TRANSVAGINAL SONOGRAPHY

TRANSVAGINAL SONOGRAPHY

Edited by

Ilan E. Timor-Tritsch, MD

Professor of Clinical Obstetrics and Gynecology
College of Physicians and Surgeons of Columbia University, New York

Director of Obstetrical and Gynecological Ultrasound
The Presbyterian Hospital in the City of New York

Associate Professor of Obstetrics and Gynecology
Technion Medical School
Deputy Director, Department of Obstetrics and Gynecology
Rambam Medical Center, Haifa, Israel

Shraga Rottem, MD

Department of Obstetrics and Gynecology
Rambam Medical Center
Haifa, Israel

Elsevier

New York · Amsterdam · London

No responsibility is assumed by the Publisher for any injury and/or damage to persons or property as a matter of products liability, negligence or otherwise, or from any use or operation of any methods, products, instructions, or ideas contained in the material herein. No suggested test or procedure should be carried out unless, in the reader's judgment, its risk is justified. Because of rapid advances in the medical sciences, we recommend that independent verification of diagnoses and drug dosages should be made. Discussions, views, and recommendations as to medical procedures, choice of drugs, and drug dosages are the responsibility of the authors.

Elsevier Science Publishing Company, Inc.
52 Vanderbilt Avenue, New York, New York 10017

Sole distributors outside the United States and Canada:
Heinemann Medical Books
22 Bedford Square, London WC1B 3HH, England

© 1988 by Elsevier Science Publishing Company, Inc.

This book has been registered with the Copyright Clearance Center, Inc.
For further information, please contact the Copyright Clearance Center, Inc.,
Salem, Massachusetts.

Library of Congress Cataloging-in-Publication Data

Transvaginal sonography.

   Includes index.
   1. Ultrasonics in obstetrics. 2. Obstetrics—
Diagnosis. I. Timor-Tritsch, Ilan E. II. Rottem,
Shraga. [DNLM: 1. Genital Diseases, Female—diagnosis.
2. Prenatal Diagnosis—methods. 3. Ultrasonic Diagnosis—
methods. WP 141 T772]
RG527.5.U48T73 1987   618.2'07'543   87-19911
ISBN 0-444-01258-3

Current printing
10 9 8 7 6 5 4

Manufactured in the United States of America

We dedicate this book to our understanding wives
Hava and Dalia
and to our children
Dafna, Orna, and Nadav

Contents

Foreword

Ultrasonography is a technology in which knowledge is rapidly being advanced by engineers and utilized by clinicians, thus changing the frontiers of knowledge and improving the quality of life for mother and fetus. If milestones in obstetrics were marked, the dramatic fall in maternal mortality probably began with the simple understanding that the spread of childbirth fever could be prevented by washing the hands. Perhaps many of the later milestones have been more technology oriented and include such events as successful cesarean births, improved surgical techniques and the use of anesthetics, blood and fluid transfusions, and, finally, the use of antibiotics.

With maternal mortality now under control, the ability to study the fetus, and even to identify the developing ovum, became possible with the introduction of ultrasonography into the specialty of obstetrics and gynecology.

If abdominal ultrasonography opened a scientific window into the womb, pelvic sonography still remained less than satisfactory. However, in this volume, through the use of vaginal ultrasonography, for the first time we see the door opened to new and exciting advances in the treatment of women.

Drs. Timor-Tritsch and Rottem have demonstrated that with use of an improved vaginal probe, now as never before, the earliest stages of human development may be visualized. Even more exciting is the application of the vaginal sonograph to the field of gynecology. Again for the first time, the lining of the fallopian tubes may be seen in a noninvasive fashion. The mature ovarian follicle can be not only identified but aspirated with the use of a vaginal probe. This procedure soon may replace anesthetic techniques and laparoscopic ovum pickup. The cervix and the uterus with their physiologic and pathologic contents may now be studied. Infections, tubal distortions, and pelvic and uterine adhesions can more easily be studied.

On the horizon exists the question whether this new technology may be used to understand and to identify earlier the growth of ovarian neoplasms, a class of malignancies that throughout this clinician's lifetime have shown little therapeutic improvement, perhaps because of delays in recognition.

It is far too early to state that this vaginal approach will become a standard of care for all gynecologists—or even reach the plateau upon which the very frequent use of ultrasonography during pregnancy exists. What is clear is that, once again, a new doorway into understanding and improved patient care has been opened.

In this book, the authors have most completely presented a wealth of visual and technical information, and given all of us an opportunity to learn and benefit from their intense studies during these past several years. The use of the vaginal probe has already been introduced into our hospital environment to teach residents and fellows, to treat patients, and to study new methods of patient care. Soon this may be another of the expected tools of patient care for all obstetricians and gynecologists.

Mortimer G. Rosen, MD
Willard C. Rappleye Professor of
Obstetrics and Gynecology and
Chairman of the Department
College of Physicians and Surgeons of
Columbia University and
The Presbyterian Hospital in the City of New York

Preface

The use of a relatively high-frequency probe through the vaginal vault for pelvic organ imaging was the product of some basic knowledge in the physics of ultrasound and the frustration of a gynecologist facing a diagnostic dilemma in a slightly obese patient suffering from a gynecological disease.

Through the last decade, the obstetrician/gynecologist has experienced a Janus-like personality. On the one hand, the "obstetrician" side of practice possessed the ability to detect intricate fetal malformations, and, lately, even to direct needles into the fetal vascular system. But the gynecology "face" was confronted with inconclusive ultrasound reports and experienced the frustration of inadequate equipment to guide the diagnostic ability available to the obstetrician.

Immediately after the ultrasonic engineers turned over to us the prototype of the first 6.5-MHz vaginal probe, we could not contain our excitement at the clarity of the pictures. They were amazingly sharp, and it was clear to all of us that we were seeing and working with something very important. Suddenly, there was no doubt about a fetal heartbeat at the end of five completed weeks from the last menstrual period in an obese patient. The developing ovarian follicles could be followed through a cycle as clearly as seeing the inside of a fruit cut through with a sharp knife. The early unruptured tubal pregnancy sprang into view and could easily be diagnosed.

Because the authors feel that these achievements are of tremendous importance to the profession, we have turned our attention to this book in order to share our techniques and results. Some of the material contained in the following pages has never before appeared in print, and we are certain that the reader will find the data as exciting as we did during the discovery. We believe that the material contained in this book represents the state of the art as we now know it, and we feel duty-bound to share this information with our colleagues.

If the diagnostic domains of early normal and abnormal pregnancy are regarded as part of the practice of gynecology rather than obstetrics, then we are rightfully entitled to consider transvaginal sonography as a major addition to gynecology. Obstetrics had its turn several years ago with the introduction of linear real-time sonography. At that time, the greatest leap forward in progress was made since the introduction of electronic and biochemical fetal monitoring. Now it is the gynecologists who are receiving attention with their new sonographic methods for diagnostic and therapeutic decision making.

The pertinent chapters will speak for themselves, but the reader must forgive us our biases when we discuss several areas we consider the ''icing on the cake.''

Undoubtedly, a closer and better look at ovarian tumors, with the potential opportunity to develop a generally used screening program for their earlier detection, may provide high-frequency transvaginal sonography with its most important role in our specialty.

Diagnosis of tubal pathology in general and early detection of tubal pregnancy in particular constitute another area in which this method has produced exciting images. If the semi-invasive transvaginal approach of treating early unruptured tubal pregnancies—saving the patient abdominal surgery and even laparoscopy (see Chapter 4)— proves to be clinically useful, we shall regard this as another outstanding achievement of transvaginal sonography.

The imaging of details of the very early pregnancy should also be mentioned here for its clinical merits as well as the potential for early recognition of the pathological pregnancy. Monitoring of follicular growth and transvaginally guided transvaginal ovum aspiration are appreciated by an increasing number of centers.

Many obstetrics and gynecology residency programs throughout the world require formal training periods in obstetrical and gynecological sonography. We speculate that within a relatively short time all departments dealing with resident training will recognize the importance of formal, hands-on training in obstetrical and gynecological ultrasonography in general, and vaginal sonography in particular. This projected rise in knowledge, together with practical experience in handling different types of transducer probes by the new generation of obstetricians and gynecologists, will necessarily bring about new methods in medical practice. If the medicolegal atmosphere can be improved by such means as excellence in practice, patient education, and education of the public at large, we envision the presence of modestly priced but clinically efficient ultrasound equipment, with its various probes, and its extensive use in each and every practice of obstetrics and gynecology. We project that the vaginal probe will be used on the spot, without much ado, as routinely as the classical vaginal speculum.

Ilan E. Timor-Tritsch
Shraga Rottem

Acknowledgments

The authors and the editors of this book would like to express their thanks to all those who made this publication possible: our secretaries Ellen Kroch and Jose Weinberg; Eli Engel, Otto Wittenberg, Bella Naphtali, and the Audiovisual Services of the College of Physicians and Surgeons, Columbia University, New York, for their assistance in preparation of the photographic material; Reba Nosoff, for reviewing, correcting, and editing the manuscript; Jane Licht and Jonathan Wiener at Elsevier Science Publishing Company, for their help and support; and, last but not least, all residents and staff members of the Department of Obstetrics and Gynecology "A" and "B" at Rambam Medical Center, for their faith in this scanning method.

Contributors

Yoram Bar-Yam, BSc
Manager, Ultrasound Probes Department, Elscint Ltd., Haifa, Israel

Dan Beck, MD
Deputy Head, Department of Obstetrics and Gynecology "A," Rambam Medical Center, Haifa, Israel

Zeev Blumenfeld, MD
Head, Reproductive Endocrinology Unit, Department of Obstetrics and Gynecology "A," Rambam Medical Center, Haifa, Israel

Rafael Boldes, MD
Resident, Department of Obstetrics and Gynecology "A," Rambam Medical Center, Haifa, Israel

Joseph M. Brandes, MD
Professor of Obstetrics and Gynecology, Technion Medical School; Director, Department of Obstetrics and Gynecology, Rambam Medical Center, Haifa, Israel

Moshe Bronshtein, MD
Department of Obstetrics and Gynecology "A," Rambam Medical Center, Haifa, Israel

Abraham Bruck, PhD
Applications Development Manager and Chief Scientist, Department of Ultrasound, Elscint Ltd., Haifa, Israel

Michael Deutsch, MD
Senior Physician, Department of Obstetrics and Gynecology "A," Rambam Medical Center, Haifa, Israel

Arieh Drugan, MD
In Vitro Fertilization Unit, Department of Obstetrics and Gynecology "A," Rambam Medical Center, Haifa, Israel

Sarit Elgali
Ultrasound Technician, Department of Obstetrics and Gynecology, Rambam Medical Center, Haifa, Israel

Yochanan Erlik, MD
Senior Physician, Department of Obstetrics and Gynecology "B," Rambam Medical Center, Haifa, Israel

Yacov Levron, MD
Resident, Department of Obstetrics and Gynecology "A," Rambam Medical Center, Haifa, Israel

Shraga Rottem, MD
Department of Obstetrics and Gynecology "A," Rambam Medical Center, Haifa, Israel

Israel Thaler, MD
Senior Physician, Department of Obstetrics and Gynecology "A," Rambam Medical Center, Haifa, Israel

Ilan E. Timor-Tritsch, MD
Professor of Clinical Obstetrics and Gynecology, College of Physicians and Surgeons of Columbia University, New York; Director of Obstetrical and Gynecological Ultrasound, The Presbyterian Hospital in the City of New York; Associate Professor of Obstetrics and Gynecology, Technion Medical School; Deputy Director, Department of Obstetrics and Gynecology, Rambam Medical Center, Haifa, Israel

CHAPTER 1

The Vaginal
Probe—Physical Considerations

Israel Thaler, MD, Abraham Bruck, PhD,
and Yoram Bar-Yam, BSc

Ultrasound is used in medical diagnosis to produce images of tissue structures from which the size and nature of the structures can be determined. For example, information concerning many types of soft-tissue organs and lesions is gathered, and the interaction of transmitted ultrasound with tissue structures gives rise to information that can be visually displayed. This information is, therefore, directly related to the acoustic, ie, ultrasonic, properties of the tissues, and is essentially different from that supplied by other diagnostic tools such as x-rays or isotope scanning.

The imaging process consists of sending short *pulses* of ultrasound into the body and using the *reflections* received from various tissues and organs to produce an image of internal structures.

Ultrasound is the term applied to mechanical pressure waves transmitted as *mechanical vibrations* through the medium. These vibrations are not random, but orderly oscillatory vibrations generated by an external source. A typical source is a crystal, electrically driven to vibrate, which is placed in contact with the outside surface of the medium. Interactions occur between the source and the particles of the surface of the medium, causing them to vibrate. These particles, in turn, cause their adjacent neighbors to start oscillating, and in a similar manner the mechanical vibrations pass very quickly through the material.

A *particle* is a small portion of the medium through which the sound travels. If the motion of a particle in a medium transmitting ultrasound is examined in detail, the particle is seen to be moving slightly back and forth parallel to the direction of wave travel. This motion is similar to that of the weight on the end of a pendulum, although the distances actually

1

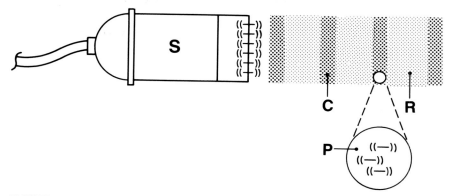

FIGURE 1.1 Formation of longitudinal waves. The vibratory motion of the source (S) forms compressions (C) and rarefactions (R). The vibrating particles (P) are similar to the weight on the end of a pendulum and vibrate along the same direction as the source motion.

moved are microscopic (in the range of one-millionth of a centimeter). Simple harmonic motion, or sinusoidal motion, is the term used here (Fig 1.1).

THE PROPERTIES OF SOUND WAVES AND IMAGE QUALITY

Like all waves, sound is described by several parameters: frequency, wavelength, propagation speed, amplitude, intensity.

Frequency is the number of complete oscillations a particle performs per second. Sound with a frequency of 20 kHz or higher is termed ultrasound, because it is beyond the frequency range of the human ear. In medical imaging, frequencies in the range 2–10 MHz are employed. The frequency of ultrasound has great influence on the image quality.

Wavelength is the length of space over which one cycle occurs, ie, the distance between any two identical points on the waveform (Fig 1.2). It plays an important role in determining ultrasonic beam widths and pulse lengths and so influences the detail (ie, resolution) obtainable in an image.

Propagation speed is the velocity of the sound wave moving through a medium. Wavelength frequency and velocity are related by

$$\text{velocity} = \text{frequency} \times \text{wavelength}$$

$$V = f \times \lambda \tag{1.1}$$

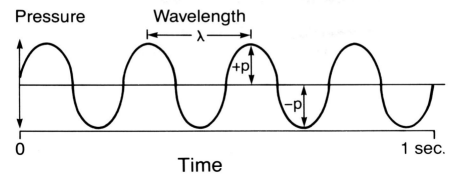

FIGURE 1.2 Wavelength (λ) and amplitude (*p*) of a wave. The frequency is four complete cycles per second, or 4 Hz.

In general, the higher the stiffness of an object, the higher the propagation speed (Table 1.1).

Propagation speed is important because imaging instruments make use of it in generating the display. If the velocity of sound in the medium is known, it is possible to calculate the wavelength using Eq. 1.1. If the average velocity of sound in tissue is assumed to be 1,540 m per second and its frequency 1 MHz, then

$$1540 = 1 \times 10^6 \times \lambda$$

Therefore

$$\lambda = 0.00154 \text{ m} = 1.54 \text{ mm}$$

TABLE 1.1 The Velocity of Ultrasound in Certain Tissues and Materials

Material	Propagation Speed (m/s)
Fat	1,450
Brain	1,540
Liver	1,550
Muscle	1,570
Soft-tissue average	1,540
Water (20°C)	1,480
Bone	4,080
Air	330

Similarly, at

2 MHz	$\lambda = 0.77$ mm
5 MHz	$\lambda = 0.31$ mm
7 MHz	$\lambda = 0.22$ mm
10 MHz	$\lambda = 0.1$ mm

This demonstrates that the higher the frequency the smaller the wavelength, and the result is better image detail.

Amplitude of an ultrasonic wave is the maximum change in pressure caused by the wave itself and is related to the intensity of the ultrasonic radiation (Fig 1.2). The greater the intensity, the greater the amplitude. The term *amplitude* is also used to describe the pulse magnitude of echoes.

Intensity is the rate at which energy flows through the unit area. This energy passes from the source to the tissue. Intensity is also defined as the power in a wave divided by the area over which the power is applied:

$$\text{intensity (W/cm}^2) = \frac{\text{power (W)}}{\text{area (cm}^2)} \qquad (1.2)$$

Intensity is expressed as watts per centimeter squared (W/cm^2).

During ultrasonic scanning, the output intensity of many instruments plays a prime role in determining the sensitivity of the instrument, that is, in determining the number and size of echoes recorded. Studies on the safety of ultrasonic techniques also require accurate knowledge of the intensities involved.

Power is the energy flow rate through the whole cross section of the beam.[1] The power is expressed in watts. For imaging of structures in close proximity to the transducer, relatively low intensities are sufficient to obtain a good-quality picture. On most instruments the intensity settings can be controlled by the user.

THE BEHAVIOR OF ULTRASONIC WAVES IN TISSUES

Diagnosis through ultrasound is accomplished by interpreting the *reflections* occurring at tissue interfaces. Short ultrasound pulses are transmitted into the region of interest, and a returning pulse or echo is generated at organ boundaries or tissue interfaces. These echoes provide rich sources of diagnostic information. An echo is generated at an interface between tissues with different acoustic properties. These properties are described as *acoustic impedance,* which is determined by the density of the tissue and the velocity of sound in that tissue:

$$\text{acoustic impedance} = \text{density} \times \text{velocity of sound}$$

$$\text{AI} = p \times v$$

(1.3)

The echo size, or intensity, is determined by the difference between the acoustic impedances of the two tissues forming the interface. The acoustic impedances of most biological tissues are so similar that only a fraction of the ultrasound is returned at each interface, most of the energy being transmitted to deeper levels. As a result, echoes from more distant (deeper) structures are also returned. This makes it possible to analyze many successive interfaces for diagnostic purposes. A notable exception is the soft tissue–bone interface. Bone has a much higher impedance than soft tissue (Table 1.2); therefore, a very strong echo is produced. The energy reflected is so large that it greatly attenuates the transmitted beam. Imaging of structures lying behind bones, therefore, becomes difficult as an *acoustic shadow* is created. Even more marked is the reflection of a gas–soft tissue interface. This makes scanning through lung or gas in the bowel impossible. In practice, gas is regarded as an impenetrable barrier that gives rise to huge echoes. When an ultrasound transducer is applied to the skin, a very thin film of air would cause a very strong attenuation of the ultrasonic beam before it even entered the body. For this reason, a coupling medium (an oil or gel) is used to provide a good sound path from the source to the skin.

As transmitted ultrasound and echoes pass through tissue, they are reduced in intensity and amplitude. This reduction in amplitude and intensity is called *attenuation*. It is due to *reflection* (described earlier), *absorption* (conversion of sound to heat), *refraction,* and *scattering*.

One result of attenuation is that echoes from structures deep within the body are much weaker than those from superficial regions. This limits the depth at which images can be obtained. Ultrasound-detecting systems

TABLE 1.2 Acoustic Impedances of Ultrasound in Certain Materials

Material	Acoustic Impedance $(g/cm^2\ s)$
Fat	1.38×10^5
Liver	1.65×10^5
Kidney	1.62×10^5
Soft-tissue average	1.63×10^5
Water (20°C)	1.48×10^5
Bone	7.80×10^5
Air	0.0004×10^5

used for diagnostic imaging are manipulated to correct this imbalance to a certain extent.

Attenuation is amplified by an increase in frequency, mainly because of a larger absorption. To give some appreciation of the role of attenuation in practice, reference is made to the thickness of tissues required to reduce intensity by half, called the *half-intensity depth*. The latter correlates with the attainable imaging depth. Half-intensity depth decreases with increased frequency and, for a given frequency, is dependent on the characteristics of the medium (Table 1.3). It can be seen from Table 1.3 that air and bone strongly attenuate the intensity of sound, whereas fluids within the body are only weakly absorbing. These fluids are often referred to as *transonic* or *translucent*. Another factor that determines echo intensity is the angle at which the ultrasonic beam strikes the reflecting surface. Because tissue interfaces are not flat, smooth reflectors, but are irregular in shape, echoes are returned even from oblique interfaces. These echoes are weaker than those reflected from perpendicular surfaces, and some may not reach the transducer face at all (Fig 1.3). In practice, complete images are obtained by varying the scanning beam direction and picking up as many reflectors (or echoes) as possible.

GENERATION OF ULTRASONIC BEAMS

An essential feature of ultrasonic instruments is the ability to produce narrow *ultrasound beams* that are highly directional. The *ultrasonic field* is a geometric description of the region encompassed by the ultrasound beam. At the high frequencies used in diagnostic ultrasound, well-di-

TABLE 1.3 Half-Intensity Depths of Various Materials in Different Frequency Ranges

Material	Half-Intensity Depth (cm)		
	2 MHz	5 MHz	10 MHz
Soft-tissue average	1.5	0.5	0.3
Blood	8.5	3	2
Water	340	54	14
Bone	0.1	0.04	—
Air	0.06	0.01	—

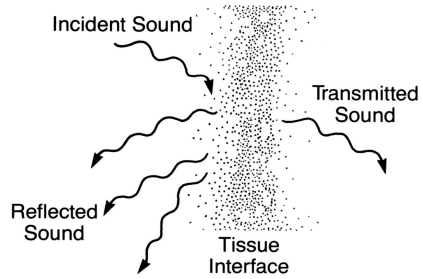

FIGURE 1.3 Reflection at a rough interface.

rected beams can be readily generated by simple devices called *ultrasonic transducers* or *probes*. Ultrasonic transducers operate on the *piezoelectricity* principle, which states that some materials (eg, ceramics, quartz) produce a voltage when deformed by an applied pressure. Piezoelectricity also results in production of a pressure when these materials are deformed by an applied voltage. As a result of both these effects, a single crystal element can be used both as a transmitter and as a receiver of ultrasonic waves. The term *transducer element* (or piezoelectric element) refers to the piece of piezoelectric material that converts electricity to ultrasound and vice versa. Typical diagnostic ultrasound transducer elements are 6–19 mm in diameter and 0.2–2 mm thick. The element and its associated case and damping and matching materials constitute the *transducer assembly* or *probe* (Fig 1.4). The damping material reduces pulse duration by damping down the vibrations. This improves axial resolution (discussed later). The matching layer facilitates sound transmission into the ·tissue. Each transducer operates at a particular frequency determined by the thickness of the transducer element and by the propagation speed of the transducer material. Source transducers can operate in two modes. The *continuous mode* is obtained by driving the transducer with a contin-

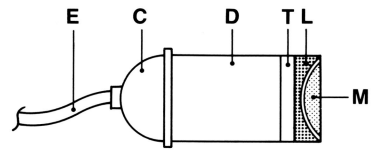

FIGURE 1.4 Structure of a basic transducer for generating pulsed ultrasound. C = case, D = damping material, E = electric cable, L = matching layer, T = transducer element, M = filler material.

uous alternating voltage; this produces alternating pressure that propagates as continuous sound waves. The *pulsed mode* is obtained by driving the transducer with voltage pulses; this produces ultrasound pulses. These transducers also convert received reflections into voltage pulses. This mode is commonly used for diagnostic ultrasound imaging.

Increasing the frequency or decreasing the number of cycles of the pulse would result in shorter spatial pulse length and, thus, better axial resolution. Damping material in the transducer probe decreases the spatial pulse length by reducing the number of cycles in each pulse.

FOCUSING OF ULTRASONIC BEAMS

Ultrasonic transducers produce narrow ultrasound beams. The shape of the beam depends primarily on the frequency and the crystal diameter for flat, unfocused transducers. The ultrasonic beam consists of two main parts: the *near zone* (or near field), which is located between the transducer and the natural focus, and the *far zone* (or far field), which is the region beyond a distance of one near-zone length (Fig 1.5). The lateral boundary of the sound field is not sharp, for the beam intensity falls off gradually with distance from the central beam axis. For improved lateral resolution (discussed later), beam diameter can be reduced by *focusing* the sound. This is accomplished by employing a curved (rather than flat) transducer element, a curved reflector, a lens, or a phased array in the probe. Focusing always occurs in the near zone. The beam diameter is decreased in the *focal region* between it and the transducer. It is widened

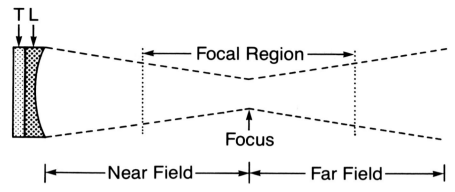

FIGURE 1.5 Focusing transducer (T) with lens (L). The focus comes closer to the transducer as the lens curvature increases, thereby shortening the near field.

in the region beyond. *Focal length* is the distance from the transducer to the center of the focal region. Most diagnostic imaging transducers are focused to some extent.

AXIAL AND LATERAL RESOLUTION

In discussing the quality of ultrasonic images, it is important to consider the fine details of the display. The basic issue is related to the minimum separation between two surfaces that gives rise to two identifiable signals. This determines the resolution attainable.

In ultrasound imaging there are two resolutions of importance: *axial* (or linear) and *lateral* (azimuthal). *Axial resolution* is the minimum reflector separation required along the direction of sound travel so that separate reflections will be produced. The important parameter in determining axial resolution is the ultrasonic pulse length (spatial pulse length):

$$\text{axial resolution} = \text{spatial pulse length}/2 \qquad (1.4)$$

Spatial pulse length can be decreased by increasing the frequency and/or reducing the number of cycles in each pulse. The latter is achieved by increasing the transducer *damping*. When damping is reduced to a minimum (ie, 2–3 cycles per pulse), the only way to improve axial resolution further is to increase frequency. Unfortunately, this possibility is also limited because attenuation increases concomitantly with frequency (see Table 1.3). The useful frequency range in medical imaging is 2 to 10 MHz because of this limitation. The closer the object of interest, the higher the frequency that can be utilized and, therefore, the better the axial resolution.

Lateral resolution is the minimum separation in the direction perpendicular to the direction of the ultrasonic beam. This is the minimal distance between two reflectors that will produce two separate reflections when the beam is scanned across them. Lateral resolution is directly proportional to the beam diameter (or width). It may be improved by reducing beam diameter, which is achieved by increasing the frequency; however, the primary means for reducing beam diameter is focusing.

THE VAGINAL ULTRASOUND PROBE

Optimal ultrasound imaging of the female pelvic organs is difficult to achieve. This is due to the pelvis being "crowded" with various structures of similar acoustic impedance (and which are, therefore, poor reflectors). The distance from the abdominal probe to these organs is relatively large, precluding the use of frequencies higher than 5 MHz. This limits both axial and lateral resolution. One method of improving image quality is by taking pelvic scans while the bladder is full. By introduction of a fluid-filled space, it is possible to observe more clearly some of the pelvic organs. Nevertheless, the problems discussed before are still present, so many fine details are missed. The concept of the vaginal probe solved many of these problems and made it possible to obtain high-quality images of the pelvic anatomy.

The main improvement is achieved by placing the ultrasonic probe closer to the pelvic structures. Most of the relevant anatomy for transvaginal imaging is within 9 cm of the vaginal fornices. This makes it possible to increase the transducer frequency up to 7 MHz while attenuation is still acceptable. Axial resolution is improved by 40–50% compared with the resolutions obtained with the conventional 3.5- to 5-MHz transducers used in abdominal scanning. Lateral resolution is also improved with the use of higher frequency, and stronger focusing is made possible by the proximity of the scanning head to the pelvic tissues.

All scans described in subsequent chapters were taken with the probe shown in Fig 1.6a. This is a mechanical sector scanner employing an oscillating transducer (Elscint ESI ED65-TV), and its dimensions are shown in Fig 1.6b. The following are some of the probe specifications:

Scan angle   Variable from 25° to 105°
Frame rate   Variable from 10 to 70 frames per second

Line density Varies according to scan angle and frame rate selected

Focal depth 4.5 cm

Resolution

    Lateral 1.3 mm

    Axial 0.5 mm

Intensity Typical rates of scan condition that give highest values:

	In Water	In Situ
Power	4.5 mW	—
SPTA	22.5 mW/cm	4.5 mW/cm
SPPA	155 W/cm	31 W/cm

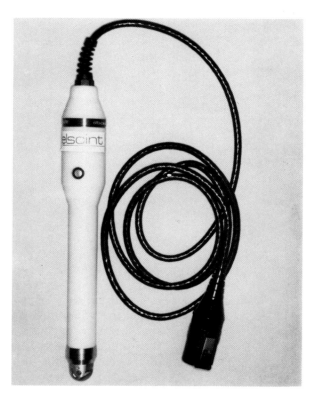

A

FIGURE 1.6 (**a**) Photograph of the vaginal probe (Elscint ESI ED65-TV).

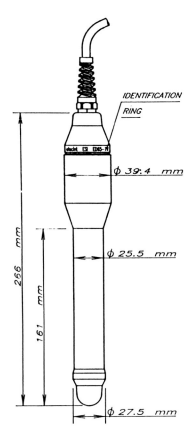

IDENTIFICATION
RING

φ 39.4 mm

φ 25.5 mm

266 mm

161 mm

φ 27.5 mm

B

FIGURE 1.6 (b) Graphic scheme of the vaginal probe showing its various dimensions.

The spatial peak pulse average intensity, *SPPA*, specifies the average intensity in a single transmitted pulse.

The spatial peak temporal average intensity, *SPTA*, specifies the intensity transmitted into one unit area, at the center of the focused beam, where intensity is maximal. This spatial peak is averaged over the time between two successive pulses. The values shown are well within the American Institute of Ultrasound in Medicine/National Electrical Manufacturers Association (AIUM/NEMA) recommendations for acceptable intensity levels for ultrasound transducers.

SUMMARY

The properties of ultrasound in tissues and the factors governing image quality were discussed. Particular emphasis was placed on the vaginal probe, which forms the basis for a "new generation" of pelvic imaging and is the main theme of this book. Only by fully understanding the properties of ultrasound can the capabilities and limitations of this technique be appreciated. A good knowledge of the basic physical principles is mandatory for the clinician as well as the investigator in attaining the highest-quality results. Much less emphasis was placed on the various technical aspects of operating ultrasound instruments, eg, machine controls, electronic image formation, scan converters, and techniques for preprocessing and postprocessing.

REFERENCES

1. Kremkau WF: Diagnostic Ultrasound: Principles, Instrumentation and Exercises. Orlando, Fla, Grune & Stratton, Inc., 1984.
2. AIUM/NEMA: Safety Standard for Diagnostic Ultrasound Equipment. Bethesda, Md, American Institute of Ultrasound in Medicine, 1981.
3. McDicken WN: Diagnostic Ultrasonics: Principles and Use of Instruments. New York, John Wiley & Sons, 1981.
4. Nyborg WL: Biophysical mechanisms of ultrasound, in Repacholi MH, Benwell DA (eds): Essentials of Medical Ultrasound. Clifton, NJ, Humana Press, 1982.
5. Powis RL, Powis WJ: A Thinker's Guide to Ultrasonic Imaging. Baltimore, Urban & Schwarzenberg, 1984.

CHAPTER 2

How Transvaginal Sonography Is Done

Ilan E. Timor-Tritsch, MD, Shraga Rottem, MD, and Sarit Elgali

The procedures for a transvaginal scan are simple and do not require special accessory equipment or space.

THE EXAMINATION TABLE

For most of the scanning procedures utilizing an "in-line" transducer probe (a probe that has an end-firing scanhead with its shaft and handle on the same axis), a flat ultrasound examining table is appropriate. If a probe with an angle between the shaft and the handle is used, however, a gynecological examination table is required. The elevated thighs enable free movement of the probe in the horizontal plane by the operator. Likewise, all surgical procedures performed by vaginal approach require a gynecological examination table having popliteal support. If a regular flat examination table is used, a special 15- to 20-cm-thick foam cushion should be inserted below the pelvis after the head and upper body of the patient are elevated. This cushion allows free movement of the examiner's hand in tilting the transducer probe in the vertical plane to achieve maximum angling.

It seems important to avoid placing the patient in the Trendelenburg position (pelvis elevated and upper body too low) since the minimal amount of pelvic fluid that is often present may help in outlining pelvic organs and, most importantly, the tubes. For this reason, we encourage the use of a slightly reversed Trendelenburg position during examination.

PREPARATION OF THE PATIENT FOR THE EXAMINATION

The first and perhaps most important prerequisite for transvaginal sonographic examination should be a thorough and complete emptying of the urinary bladder, for three reasons: (1) a full bladder may "occupy" most of the screen and displace important "target organs" to be scanned; (2) sound waves passing through the bladder filled with a low-impedance fluid create the well-known effect of *enhancement* (this high-echo area below the bladder interferes with a proper gain setting); (3) a full bladder distorts pelvic anatomy by compressing pelvic organs and displacing possible ovarian or tubal pathology beyond the reach of the transducer.

A thorough bimanual pelvic examination and/or a transabdominal–transvesical ultrasound examination may provide the gynecologist with additional valuable information. These two examinations should therefore precede the transvaginal ultrasound examination.

A short explanation of the procedure will prevent patient anxiety. Most patients do not associate ultrasound scanning with a *vaginal* examination; therefore, it is necessary to inform the patient about this relatively "new way" of performing sonographic examination. One should mention the similarity between the vaginal transducer and the familiar vaginal speculum the patient has surely experienced before.

THE EQUIPMENT AND THE TRANSDUCER

The ultrasound equipment should be prepared before the transducer is introduced into the vagina. Patient identification should be typed in through the keyboard and the screen made ready for work. Additional recording equipment should be prepared and switched to "standby" mode. This will reduce the time of the actual vaginal examination. The transducer tip is then covered with transducer gel and introduced into a protective rubber sheet. This may be a plain surgical rubber glove. One of the "fingers" is used and firmly pulled over the tip of the probe to avoid trapping air, which creates unwanted artifacts on the screen. The covered transducer probe is then dipped in transducer gel to facilitate vaginal penetration.

Schwimmer et al[1] have recommended caution in employing the commonly used ultrasound coupling gels for vaginal transducer lubrication in patients who will undergo insemination immediately after transvaginal examination. Some of the most commonly used coupling gels were found to affect sperm motility adversely.

At or close to midcycle, when this may become relevant, the cervix ordinarily produces enough mucus to enable a good sound coupling between the transducer probe and the vaginal vault. It is, therefore, technically feasible to perform a vaginal scan at midcycle without artificially lubricating the tip of the probe.

Some manufacturers market special rubber or plastic sheets to cover the transducer probe. Others suggest the use of inexpensive condoms to protect the probe and maintain aseptic conditions during scanning.

After insertion of the transducer probe, the required gain curve and magnification are selected to obtain the best possible image on the screen.

To obtain images in various directions, planes, and depths, three main manipulations of the probe are possible: (1) tilting or angling the shaft by its handle so as to point the tip of the probe in any direction in the pelvis; (2) pushing–pulling the whole probe to bring a deeper or a closer organ into the focal region or actually into the focal length; (3) rotating the handle slowly along the longitudinal axis of the probe to change the scanning plane along a 360° range. Figures 2.1a–2.1c illustrate the above-discussed scanning planes and directions achieved by the examiner.

In addition to these manual manipulations of the probe, the symmetrically end-firing "fan" of the beam can be tilted in an off-axis scanning direction by the appropriate electronic controls. Thus, scanning of the whole pelvis is possible. Most transvaginal transducer probes utilize a symmetrically end-firing probe with various scanning angles from 90° to 240°. Other probes use an inbuilt, fixed upward tilt of the scanning plane in addition to a second angle between the handle and the shaft carrying the transducer itself. The properties, specifications, and possibilities of the different transducers should always be examined in advance by the potential buyer.

THE EXAMINATION

The first structure on the path of the vaginal probe to its final place of scanning the pelvis is the cervix. If the cervix has to be scanned it may be done as the probe penetrates 2.5–3 cm into the vagina, 2–3 cm before the tip of the probe reaches the cervix itself. This prevents the picture from being obscured by air that may be trapped in the fornices at the end of a prolonged or a repeated examination. The cervix may also be examined after locating the uterus and then pulling the probe slowly outward. One should always obtain a horizontal and a vertical plane (Fig 2.2) in which the central structure to be visualized is the cervical canal. Cystic structures adjacent to the cervical canal and external os are frequently seen.

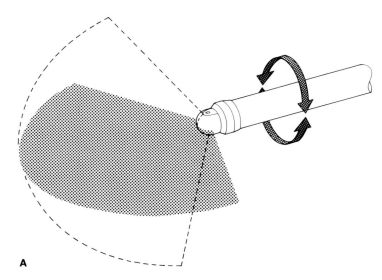

A

FIGURE 2.1 Basic scanning directions, planes, and depths achieved by moving the probe. Any combination of the following may be used to obtain the best possible image: (**a**) rotating the probe along its longitudinal axis; (**b**) angling the shaft, pointing it in any desired direction; (**c**) pushing or pulling the probe, "positioning" deeper or closer structures within the focal range of the transducer.

They represent endocervical cysts and Nabothian cysts. Cervical pregnancy should always be kept in mind and looked for if ectopic pregnancy is suspected, but other pathology of the cervix is of course more prevalent.

The most prominent landmark in the pelvis is usually the *uterus*. If the uterus is detected on the screen the routine examination should start systematic scanning. One should start scanning from the back to the front using the horizontal plane first. If the uterus is anteverted and anteflexed, the first cross section to be seen is the cervix. A slow upward scan will reveal the body and finally the fundus of the uterus. With the same sequence (scanning from the back to the front) in a retroverted uterus, the fundus is visualized first and the cervix last. The transverse or horizontal scan should be followed by the vertical scanning plane, which will reveal the entire uterus with its endometrial lining (Fig 3.6, p 33). Scanning of the lateral uterine margin on either side may reveal the ingoing, outgoing, and pulsating vascular packets at the level of the junction between the cervix and the body of the uterus (Fig 3.5, p 32). Blood flow is readily seen in these vessels with this high-frequency transducer. Blood flow measurements of the uterine artery and vein may be done using this site.

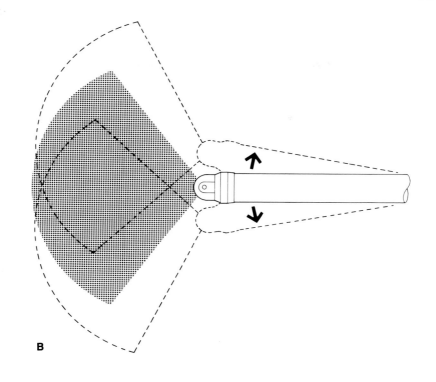

B

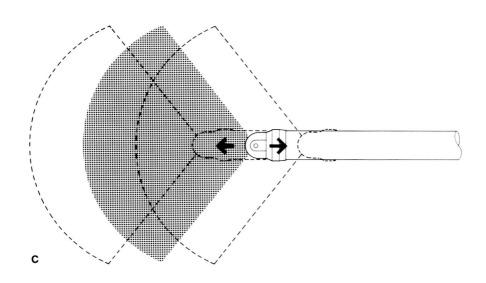

C

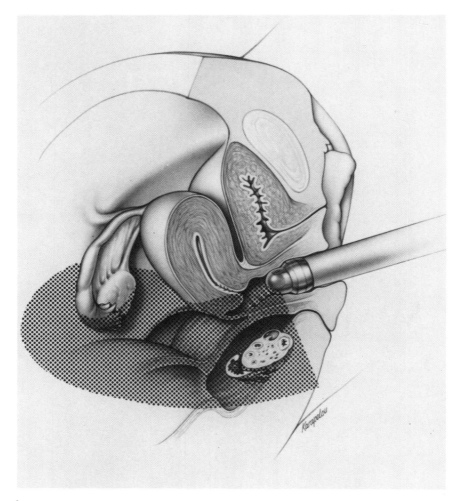

A

FIGURE 2.2 The anatomical relation to the transvaginally inserted probe and the pelvic organs demonstrates (**a**) the horizontal scanning plane, and (**b**) the vertical, or sagittal, scanning plane.

After the uterus and its contents are examined, the *pouch of Douglas* should be sought. In many cases there is some fluid present in the cul-de-sac. This minimal amount of fluid may be detected. Free fluid outlines the posterior wall of the uterus and sometimes even the ovaries. As mentioned before, it is disadvantageous to place the patient in the Trendelen-

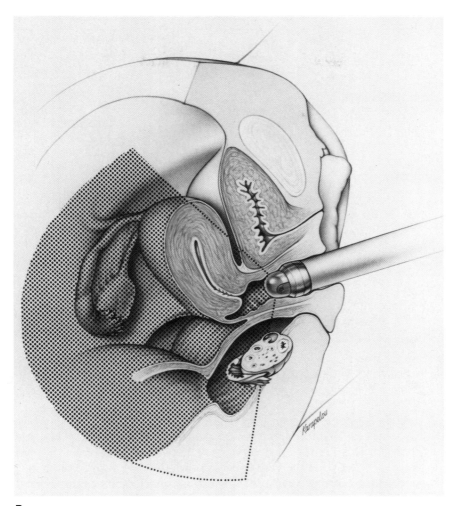

B

burg position, since some of the fluid will spill from the pouch of Douglas to other lower-lying spaces. Because of the high resolution of the pictures, even a small amount of fluid in the cul-de-sac may impress the novice sonographer, leading to a false interpretation, namely of "a large fluid collection" (Fig 2.3).

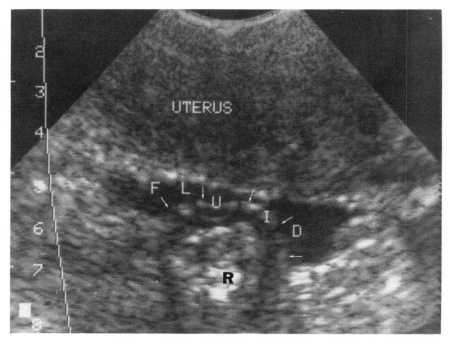

FIGURE 2.3 A small amount (approximately 5–8 mL) of pelvic fluid is present in the cul-de-sac, behind the uterus. A cross section of the rectum (R) and its peritoneal cover (arrows) is visible.

Figure 2.4 comprises images of the iliac vein and artery. They are easily located by pointing the transducer tip to the side of the pelvis and searching for them in the transverse as well as the vertical plane. Blood flow is seen in the vein; the vein appears medially and closer to the pelvic organs than the common iliac artery, which lies in a lateral position, is half the size of the vein, and pulsates passively, moving the adjacent vein. These two large vessels are of great importance as the lateral landmarks of the pelvis during the sonographically guided removal of oocytes since the ovaries are sometimes in very close proximity (even adherent) to the peritoneum covering them.

The tip of the transducer probe should now be pointed toward the side of the uterus to visualize the adnexa. The *ovaries* are the most prominent landmarks of the adnexa. They are distinct because of their relatively lower echogenic texture as well as the different-sized Graafian follicles. The follicles appear as echo-free, translucent, round structures from several millimeters to 2 cm in diameter. During the reproductive years, these

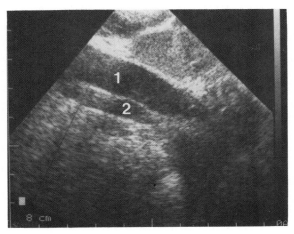

FIGURE 2.4 Right iliac vein (**1**) and artery (**2**). Pulsation of the artery was seen in real time.

follicles serve as sonographic "markers" of the ovaries. After menopause it is hard to find the ovaries because the above-described "markers" (ie, the follicles) are not present and the ovaries themselves undergo atrophy. If the ovaries are visualized in the postmenopausal patient, this should be clearly mentioned in the sonographic report and a workup of the case is advisable.

If the uterus and the ovaries are localized, the *tubes* may be scanned. They should be sought under the imaginary horizontal plane drawn at the level of the endometrial line at the sides of the uterus. If found, they are usually behind the ovaries or in the cul-de-sac. If they are normal and healthy or no fluid surrounds them, they cannot be visualized. If pathological (eg, dilated, thick, fluid-filled, or housing a gestational sac), they are usually outstanding and easily recognized.

The next step is to look for *space-occupying lesions* in the pelvis. Since there is no specific place to direct our attention, the entire pelvis must be systematically "covered" by imaginary horizontal and vertical coordinates, and a thorough search should be made along these planes.

Reminder. The effective focal zone of the 6.5-MHz transducer ends at 7–8 cm. One may diagnose structures deeper than 8 cm, but they appear "blurred" and are irregularly outlined. A fairly large mass may be missed by vaginal scanning if, because of its size, it does not extend deep enough into the pelvis. If a pelvic mass has to be ruled out or is suspected, an additional transabdominal scan should be performed.

SPECIAL MANEUVERS THAT MAY BE EMPLOYED

The examiner may place the other hand on the lower abdomen to bring pelvic structures closer to the tip of the probe, as in a regular bimanual pelvic–abdominal examination.

In case of pelvic pain, localization of the point of maximal intensity under direct vision and gentle pressure with the tip of the transducer probe may be attempted.

Diagnosis of pelvic adhesions becomes possible by the *"sliding organs sign"*: The transducer tip is pointed at the uterus, ovaries, or any pelvic finding (eg, ovarian mass, tubo-ovarian complex), and a gentle push–pull movement of several centimeters is started. If no adhesions are present, the organs will move freely in the pelvis. This displacement of organs is perceived on the screen as a sliding movement. One may, for instance, observe the free sliding of an ovarian mass over the lateral wall of the pelvis, which of course is static. In the case of a tubo-ovarian complex, the relative locations of the uterus, tube, and ovary will not change under the pushing motion of the probe, because of extensive adhesions preventing normal and physiological sliding of these organs.

If, during bimanual pelvic–abdominal examination, a palpable finding is obvious, one may perform a *one-finger* vaginal examination and introduce the probe along this finger, directing it at the finding in question. This makes palpable findings instantly "visible."

Sometimes the region of interest is very *close* to the transducer; thus, a disturbed and unclear picture appears on the screen. In this case, the transducer should be pulled outward 1 or 2 cm until the picture clears. This procedure may help if the cervix is examined. If the far end of the picture is blurred, the transducer is pushed gently into the vagina until a "sharper" picture is obtained. Both maneuvers are based on bringing the region of interest into the focal area of the transducer. To end the scanning, the probe should be pulled out slowly from the vagina with constant observation of the screen. At times, new and heretofore undetected findings may be revealed.

THE REPORT

After transvaginal sonographic examination, a detailed report must be issued. This report is different from that generated after transabdominal–pelvic sonography. The increased diagnostic power of transvaginal sonography imposes a higher demand on the sonographer. *Detection* or *lack of detection* of the ovaries, tubes, or fluid in the Douglas space and early demonstration of the presence or the absence of an intrauterine or extrauterine pregnancy should, therefore, be explicitly mentioned in the report. In the next chapters, transvaginal sonography of the pelvis and pelvic organs is described in detail.

REFERENCE

1. Schwimmer SR, Rothman CM, Lebovic J, et al: The effect of ultrasound coupling gels on sperm motility in vitro. Fertil Steril 1984;42(6):946–947.

CHAPTER 3

Scanning the Uterus

Ilan E. Timor-Tritsch, MD, Shraga Rottem, MD,
and Rafael Boldes, MD

The normal uterus is the largest midline structure in the pelvis. It should
first be scanned in the transverse (horizontal) plane, from the back to the
front. The transducer tip should be pointed toward the sacrum. Scanning
in the longitudinal (vertical) plane should follow. The transverse and longitudinal scanning planes are not always identical to the transverse and
longitudinal planes of the specific pelvic organ (eg, the longitudinal section of a uterus displaced by an adnexal mass is different from that of the
pelvis).

Systematic scanning of the uterus should start with the cervix followed by the body, then the cavity, and finally the space posterior to it,
namely, the cul-de-sac. Special attention should be given to evaluation of
the uterus in the postmenopausal period as well as in cases of suspected
uterine malformations.

EXAMINATION OF THE CERVIX

If the uterus is anteverted and the scanning is done in the transverse
plane, the first structure to appear on the screen is the cervix. If a retroverted uterus is present, the transducer will first reveal the fundus of the
uterus, which, in this case, is close to the sacrum. Scanning in the longitudinal plane will easily reveal the exact position of the uterus and the
cervix in the pelvis.

The vaginal portion of the cervix with the external os may be examined. Nabothian cysts of different size may appear as translucent, ex-

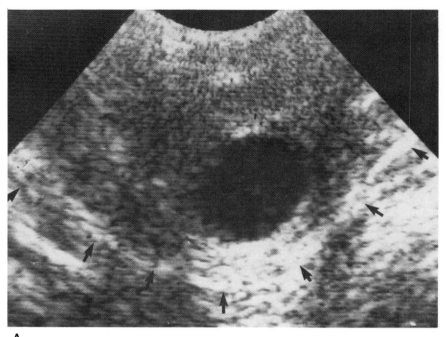

A

FIGURE 3.1 (**a**) Cross section of the cervix close to the external os. The 9 × 11-mm Nabothian cyst (confirmed by speculum examination) is situated in the posterior lip, which is delineated by small arrows. (**b**) Longitudinal section of the same Nabothian cyst shown at a smaller scale. Note endometrium on the left side (thick arrow). The external os is on the right side, approximately near the open arrow. The posterior aspect of the uterus is outlined by small black arrows.

tremely thin-walled round structures (Figs 3.1a and 3.1b). The cervix should be examined using the vertical plane as well, by turning the transducer plane 90°. This will cause the endocervical canal to become the most prominent structure on the screen. Sometimes, cystic formations of various sizes (0.5–3 cm) may appear along the endocervical canal. These probably represent dilated (obstructed?) endocervical glands, not yet described in the literature dealing with ultrasound.

The most important differential diagnosis of this finding may be the extremely remote possibility of a very early cervical pregnancy (diagnostic studies of this clinical entity by transvaginal sonography [TVS] are not yet completed).

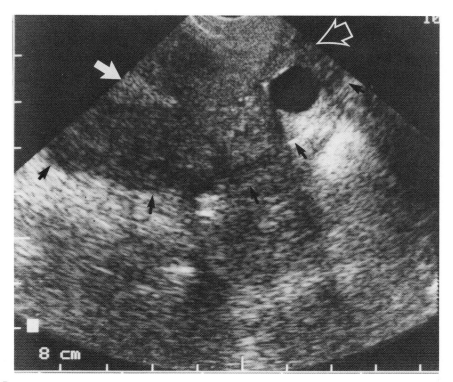

B

In most cases it is possible to visualize the cervix on a longitudinal view. The external and internal os as well as the cervical canal should be inspected and measurements taken. The internal cervical os is more distinct in the pregnant than in the nonpregnant uterus (Figs 3.2, 3.3, and 3.4).

Examination of the cervix in a pregnant patient with vaginal spotting or slight bleeding may be controversial. "Clinically," any kind of vaginal manipulation or examination is contraindicated in these cases. One should, however, remember the basic technique employed to examine the cervix: the tip of the probe is 3–4 cm away from the external os so that it can be adequately seen and captured in the effective focal range of the

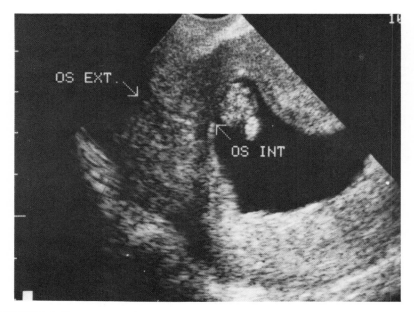

FIGURE 3.2 The normal uterine cervix of a 14-week-pregnant patient.

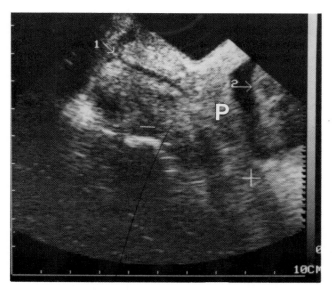

FIGURE 3.3 The placenta previa (p) overlying the internal cervical os. The external os (1) is visible. Part of the fetus (2) is also shown in this section.

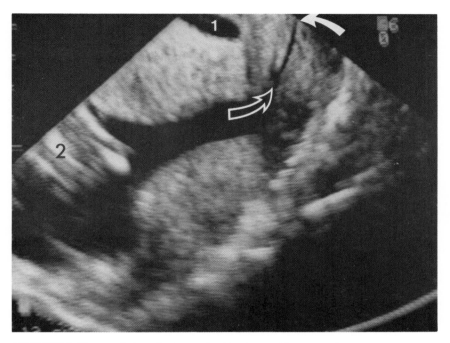

FIGURE 3.4 The cervix is pointing up in this picture. The normal cervical canal (2 mm in diameter) is imaged through its entire length (23 mm) from the external os (white arrow) to the internal os (open arrow). The maternal bladder (1) adjacent to the cervix is shown. Part of the fetal body (2) is on the left side surrounded by amniotic fluid. Image blurring is due to the photograph having been taken from the replay of a videorecorded picture.

transducer. If this basic rule is kept in mind, consideration may be given to the careful use of transvaginal sonography (TVS) in cases of pregnancy-related vaginal bleeding. This view is reinforced by the fact that a full bladder at the time of transabdominal scanning (which is a logical and established alternative) in cases of a suspected placenta previa may result in a false-positive diagnosis.

For the first time we may have the opportunity and the right tool to make direct observations and study the entity called "cervical incompetence." It still seems premature to draw clinical conclusions based on this new route of cervical scanning before more extensive descriptions of the normal and abnormal cervix, with or without the presence of an intrauterine pregnancy, are available.

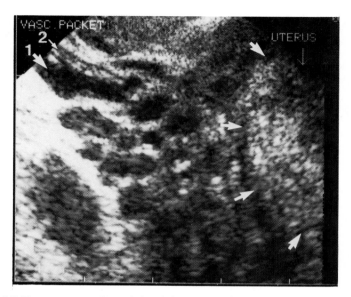

FIGURE 3.5 Transverse section of the right parametrium at the level of the internal cervical os. The vascular packet consists of the uterine vein (1) and artery (2), as well as the rich vascular web approaching the uterus (outlined by small arrows) of which only a portion is included in this scan.

During or after examination of the cervix, approximately at the level of the internal os, close to the lateral aspect of the cervix, an abundant packet of blood vessels may be recognized (Fig 3.5). Blood flow is clearly seen on real-time scanning. The two major vessels, the uterine artery and vein, are outstanding and quite easily recognized. Flow measurements in these vessels may be performed at this site.

THE UTERINE BODY

Several aspects should be considered:

First, the position of the uterus should be determined. A simple rule can be applied. If, on the longitudinal (vertical) plane, the cavity line is concave ("bulging" downward), the uterus is anteverted (Fig 3.6a). If the cavity line is convex and its "fundal end" points forward (the cavity line

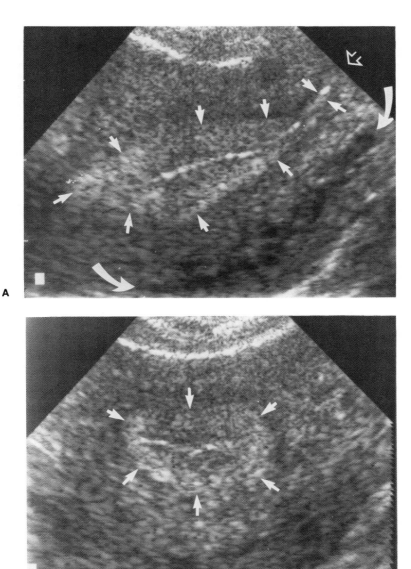

FIGURE 3.6 (**a**) Longitudinal section of an anteverted uterus. The endometrium is outlined by arrows. The discrete cavity line is normal in appearance. The cervix is on the right side of the picture (open arrow). Note the sonolucent, vascular space extending along the imaginary line connecting the two white curved arrows. Flow in them was seen in real time. They most probably represent the arcuate uterine vessels. (**b**) Transverse section of the same uterus. The patient was in her midcycle.

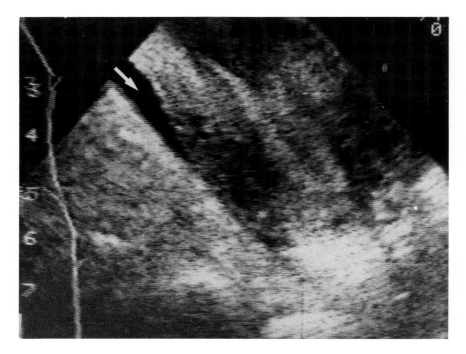

FIGURE 3.7 Longitudinal section of a retroverted uterus. A small amount of fluid is present in the cul-de-sac (arrow) after ovulation has taken place.

is "bulging" upward), the uterus is retroverted (Fig 3.7). The uterus is usually in a midline position. If scanned in the transverse plane any lateral displacement of the uterine body (by an adnexal mass or by adhesions) should be noted and described.

Second, the uterine body should be screened for the most frequent pathology of the myometrium: the uterine leiomyoma and fibroid, which vary in size and location. Their sonographic appearance is typical: variable echogenicity arranged in bundlelike "turbulent" structures interspersed with acoustic shadows generated by dense fibroid tissue (Fig 3.8). The echogenic and echo-free bundlelike structures observed on the screen resemble the classical low-power microscopic picture of the fibroids with their bundles of fibrocyte-containing stroma and muscular layers. One wonders if this 6.5-MHz transducer producing high-resolution

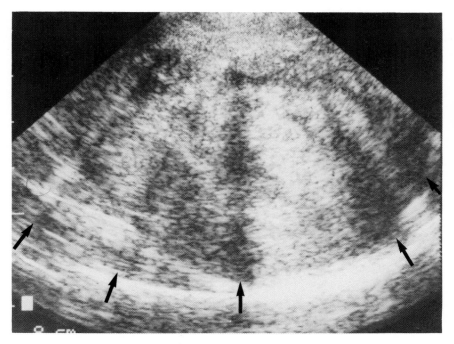

FIGURE 3.8 Typical TVS picture of a diffusely fibroid uterus. Irregular echogenicity and acoustic shadows (marked by arrows) alternate in an enlarged uterus.

pictures may be the first step in a future high frequency–high resolution sonographic tissue definition.

Often a decision must be made as to the exact nature of a mass adjacent to the uterus. The most prevalent problem is whether the mass originates in the ovary or is contiguous with the uterus (fibroid). In these cases the possible interface between the two structures should be carefully scrutinized. The "sliding organs sign" described in Chapter 2 may help in diagnosing a freely moving ovarian mass. If the solid mass moves together and in the same direction when pushed with the probe and if the sonographic texture is similar to that of the uterus, a diagnosis of a fibroid can tentatively be made (Fig 3.9).

A small intramural myoma can easily be detected and its exact location evaluated (Fig 3.10).

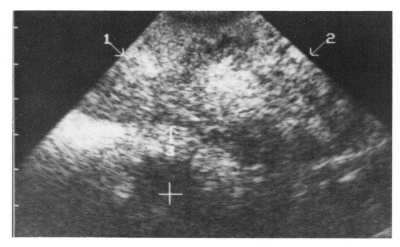

FIGURE 3.9 A 3 × 4-cm fibroid (1) arising from the right wall of the uterus (2). The wide basis of the fibroid as well as the similar sonographic structure makes it possible to establish this diagnosis by TVS.

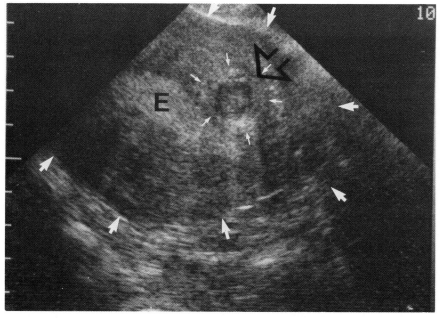

FIGURE 3.10 Longitudinal uterine section. The uterus is outlined by the large white arrows. The endometrium (E) is distorted by the 1 × 1.6-cm intramural fibroid (open black arrow) outlined by the small white arrows.

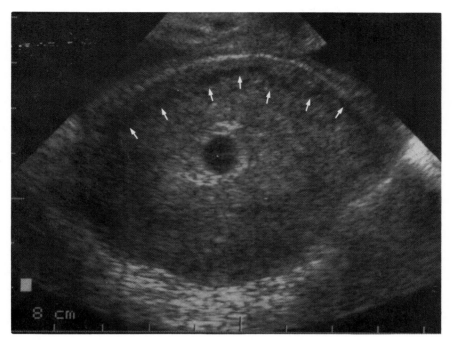

FIGURE 3.11 This transvaginal sonogram was taken during hysterosalpingography. The injected fluid distends the cavity, which seemed to be devoid of gross pathology. Note the vascular spaces in the myometrium of the anterior wall (arrows).

At times, "cavity formation" resulting from central necrosis is detected in a fibroid. These cavities contain a sonolucent material and could be misdiagnosed as gestational sacs. The true gestational sac is recognized by its well-known sonographic characteristics and, therefore, differentiated from a degenerative process within a large fibroid.

With careful scanning, we were able to detect, in almost all uteri of women of reproductive age, a vascular plexus located in the myometrium, extending almost parallel and at a constant depth of about 1 cm from the visceral peritoneum (Figs 3.6a and 3.11). Flow was noted in this space.

Third, the postmenopausal (usually atrophic) uterus is worth mentioning here. It is significantly smaller and is seldom anteverted and anteflexed. The atrophic but disease-free uterus has a uniform echogenicity (Fig 3.12); its endometrial lining is hard to differentiate from a myometrial

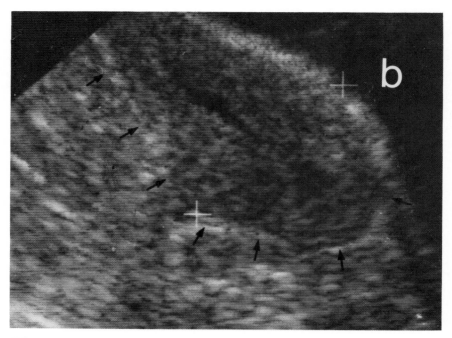

FIGURE 3.12 The atrophic uterus (4.2 × 2.2 × 2.5 cm) of a postmenopausal patient is outlined by the anteriorly situated bladder (b) and the small arrows. The cavity is filled with a small amount of fluid. No vaginal bleeding was evident in this patient.

structure or is extremely thin (Fig 3.13). The possibility of detecting an endometrial polyp in an atrophic uterus was mentioned above (Fig 3.14).

Fourth, evaluation of the uterine cavity and its endometrial lining is the next step of the scanning. A normal and "empty" uterus shows a regular, thin, and obvious "cavity line." This should be evident on longitudinal as well as serial transverse sections (Fig 3.6). The sonographic appearance of the endometrium changes through the menstrual cycle. This cyclic change is discussed in detail in Chapter 9. Because of the inherent high resolution of this transducer, the endometrial grading appears easier to perform by TVS.

The most common contents of the uterine cavity are the products of conception. Two chapters are devoted to this entity (see Chapters 6 and 7).

In the case of excessive menstrual bleeding, the endometrial lining

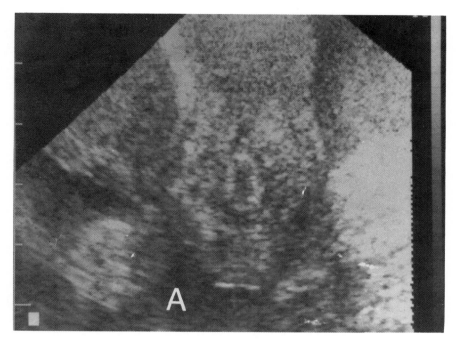

FIGURE 3.13 The atrophic retroverted uterus (5.0 × 2.5 × 2.5 cm) is surrounded by ascitic fluid (A) and several pelvic masses. On the basis of TVS, an endometrial origin of the malignancy was excluded by the sonographer. The report of the pathologist was adenocarcinoma of the ovary.

apparently becomes thin, and the blood-filled cavity is well outlined (Fig 3.15). Artificially injected fluid can serve as "ultrasonic contrast material" to outline possible endometrial or other space-occupying structures that disrupt the normal anatomy of the uterine cavity (Fig 3.11).

A large enough endometrial polypoid structure may be detected by TVS. If uterine bleeding also occurs, the outline of an intracavital structure becomes more obvious (Fig 3.14).

The cul-de-sac is anatomically related and adjacent to the uterus and, therefore, is mentioned mainly in this chapter. If there is no fluid in this pouch, it is hard to visualize; only a few milliliters of pelvic fluid outline this space clearly (Figs 3.7 and 2.3). Larger amounts of fluid are hard to miss (Figs 3.16 and 5.3). In cases of ascites, the peritoneal surface of the uterus (Fig 3.17) and the pelvis (Fig 5.13) can be examined for adhesions and irregularities.

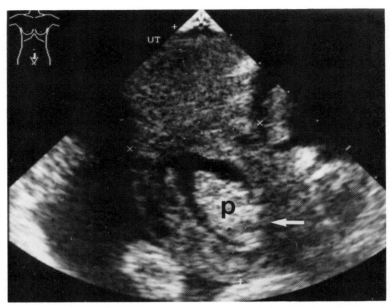

FIGURE 3.14 The atrophic uterus (6.5 × 3.2 × 2.8 cm) of a 53-year-old patient is surrounded by pelvic fluid (ascites). The cavity is filled with fluid outlining a 2 × 1.2 × 1.4-cm polypoid structure (p) emerging from the upper anterior wall (arrow). The anterior wall is not outlined and seems to be contiguous with an irregular mass. The scan was performed with a 5-MHz transvaginal probe (General Electric).

The dilated and fluid-filled hydrosalpinx is sometimes found in the cul-de-sac. If intraperitoneal bleeding is present, as in the case of a ruptured corpus luteum or tubal gestation, blood clots may form in this space. These can be diagnosed if unclotted blood surrounds the irregularly echogenic clots (Fig 8.9), which move from side to side if the patient tilts her pelvis from side to side during the examination.

If one is in doubt about the exact nature of pelvic fluid visible by TVS, a transvaginal sonographically guided needle-puncture can be easily—but more important, reliably—done to aspirate some of this fluid for identification.

Malformations of the uterus are easily detected. Despite the fact that only images of a bicornuate uterus (Fig 3.18) and a septum within a pregnant uterus (Fig 3.19) are presented here, it would appear that these constitute only a fraction of all possible uterine malformations.

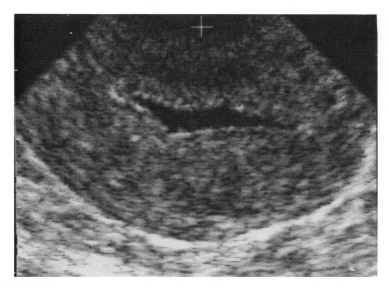

FIGURE 3.15 Transverse scan of a patient with menorrhagia on the third menstrual day. Note the thin endometrial lining as well as the sonolucent blood in the cavity.

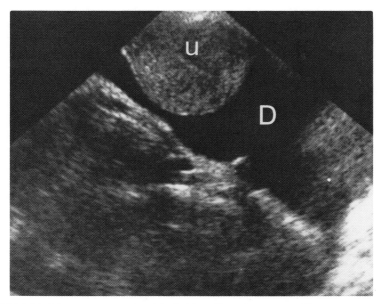

FIGURE 3.16 A large amount of pelvic fluid outlines the pouch of Douglas (D) and the normal uterus (u).

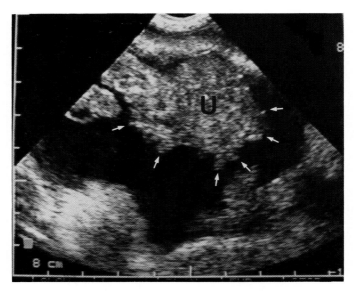

FIGURE 3.17 Ascites in a patient with tuberculotic peritonitis. Note the irregular surface of the uterus (u) "floating" in the fluid. The irregular uterine surface may result from the fibrin deposits (arrows) prevalent in this disease. No direct visual proof could be obtained in this case.

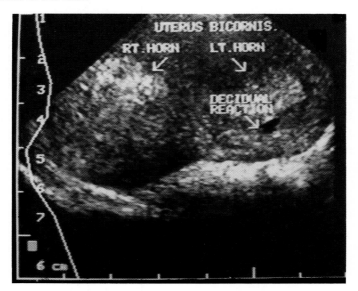

FIGURE 3.18 Transverse section of a bicornuate uterus. The right and left horns can be recognized by their separate endometrial linings. Pregnancy and, subsequently, a spontaneous abortion were diagnosed in the left horn.

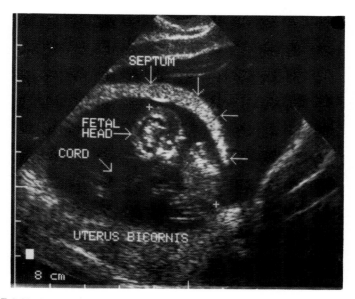

FIGURE 3.19 A pregnant septate uterus is scanned. The septum is well delineated. A normal 9-week 5-day fetus is seen on the left side.

Sonographic pictures of cervical and endometrial cancer were not yet available at the time of this writing. These entities undoubtedly present a wide field for descriptive transvaginal sonography. Evaluation continues on the role of TVS in the diagnosis and follow-up of cervical as well as endometrial malignancy. In conclusion, the authors consider TVS the primary sonographic approach to rule in or rule out uterine pathology.

CHAPTER 4

The Fallopian Tubes

Ilan E. Timor-Tritsch, MD, Shraga Rottem, MD, and Yacov Levron, MD

Ultrasonic evaluation of the Fallopian tubes presents one of the greatest challenges for the sonographer. Regardless of the technology applied, only gross pathology may be recognized and described. The available literature regarding the use of sonography in tubal diagnosis is scarce and limited to the description of tubal pregnancy and the gross, fluid-filled tubes. It was the clinician's responsibility to translate the sonographic report of a "fluid-filled adnexal mass" into a practical clinical diagnosis. The list of differential diagnoses could not usually be shortened substantially on the grounds of such a sonographic report.

The main reasons for the inability to see the normal tube or to partially view the fluid-filled tube are multiple. *First,* and probably most important, is the use of 3.5- or 5.0-MHz transducers. These transducers achieve adequate sound penetration when applied through the abdominal wall and the distended bladder; however, a price is paid in terms of resolution for the adequate penetration and relatively low attenuation that are achieved.

Because of the physical limitations of the 3.5- and 5.0-MHz transducers, axial and lateral resolution is limited to a relatively coarse outline of the general pelvic anatomy and pathology. This is even more the case if the delicate tubal anatomy and pathology are considered.

Second, the normal Fallopian tube is a poor sonic reflector itself, devoid of clear interfaces (eg, fluid/tissue) that would produce a clear organ outline. It may now be easier to understand why transabdominal sonography does not produce sufficiently clear images of the healthy or the diseased Fallopian tube.

45

It also may now seem more logical that a transvaginal probe using a higher-frequency transducer crystal should overcome the above-mentioned limitations. The sound wave, on its way to the closer pelvic organs (in this case the tubes), would be less attenuated; therefore, because of the higher frequency employed, an image with a higher-frequency resolution is obtained.

THE NORMAL TUBE

The healthy Fallopian tube usually cannot be visualized unless some type of surrounding fluid is present. Such "contrasting" fluid may be the following:

1. The normal serous pelvic fluid present in a significant number of healthy women[1] amounting to several milliliters (Fig 4.1).
2. Follicular fluid released at midcycle through the ovulation process, reaching 4–10 mL; therefore, at times of presumed ovulation or shortly thereafter the chances of detecting the ampullar part (Fig 4.2) and the fimbrial end (Fig 4.3) are increased.
3. Blood in various quantities.

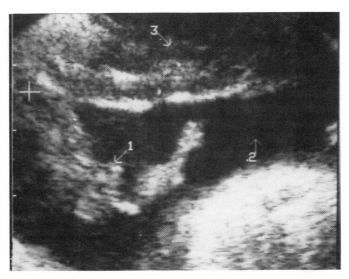

FIGURE 4.1 The distal end of the normal left tube (1) freely floating in fluid (2) below the uterus (3). The patient complained of pelvic pain.

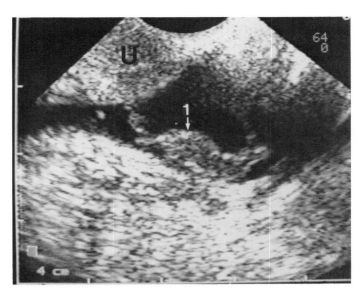

FIGURE 4.2 Clearly seen is the ampullar part of the left tube (1) surrounded by fluid in the pelvis; u = uterus.

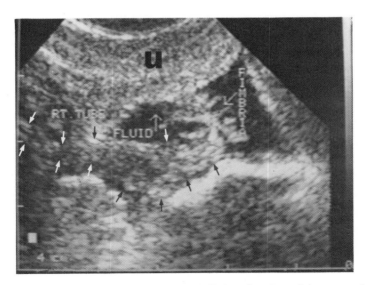

FIGURE 4.3 The same patient as in Figure 4.2. Below the uterus (u), surrounded by a physiological amount of fluid in the Douglas space, the right tube, including the ampullar part with the delicate fimbrial end, is imaged.

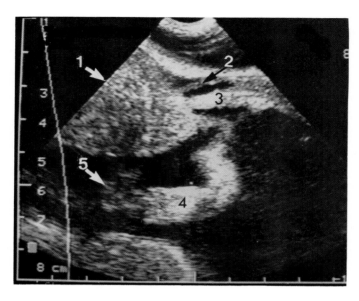

A

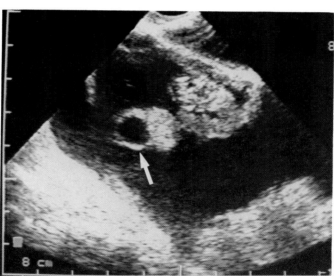

B

FIGURE 4.4 (a) Massive ascites outlines the uterus (1), round ligament (2), broad ligament (3), and left tube (4) with fimbrial end (5). **(b)** In the same patient, the left tube is imaged. A small 1-cm morgagnian cyst is seen at the fimbrial end (arrow).

4. Ascitic fluid usually produced by a neoplastic, obstructive, vascular, or other rare condition.

5. The products of an exudative or infectious process (Fig 4.4).

If the patient is being examined in a slightly reversed Trendelenburg position, advantage can be taken of even the minute amount of fluid that will be pooled in the pelvis. Fluid, as previously mentioned, is the best acoustic interface for tubal imaging.

A recent study[1] pointed out that regardless of ovulation inhibition a small amount of pelvic fluid was found in female patients in the reproductive years. This fluid increased in volume at and immediately after mid-cycle.

If detected, the tube presents as a tortuous echogenic structure about 1 cm wide; however, on the screen its width may vary along its entire length because of the two-dimensional scanning plane "cutting through" different parts of the "undulating" tube (Fig 4.2). The tubal lumen can be discerned only if it is filled with fluid, and when enough fluid is present, the fimbrial end of the tube may be seen (Fig 4.3). Pathological amounts of pelvic fluid enable imaging of the normal or abnormal salpinx. If the tube is detected, longitudinal and serial cross sections should be made by rotating the probe around its longitudinal axis. One advantage of the transvaginal probe is the possibility of measuring the uterus, the ovaries, and the tube with a push–pull motion of the probe. This light pressure may move the tube into various positions to improve imaging.

The *affected tube* is diagnosed by examining its wall, luminal contents, and adherence to its surroundings.

The *tubal wall* may be evaluated if its lumen is filled with contrasting fluid. If, in addition, free fluid coats the salpinx, the wall will be even better defined.

An *acute* disease such as an inflammatory process or tubal gestation usually leads to thickening of the wall (Figs 4.5–4.8). During this acute stage the longitudinal endosalpingeal folds can be visualized (Figs 4.7 and 4.8). A tortuous hydrosalpinx is shown in Figure 4.6; this uniformly thickened wall with a total flattening of the endosalpinx may represent a transition to the *chronic* hydrosalpinx, which is characterized by a stretched, thin wall (Fig 4.9). In two patients with long histories of pelvic inflammatory disease and infertility, in addition to a fluid-filled, dilated tube, small nodular structures of the wall were detected. The nodules appeared as spaced beads on a string (Fig 4.9). Speculation had it that they were the remnants of the longitudinal endosalpingeal folds of the diseased mucosa. The diagnosis of hydrosalpinx was documented in these cases by laparoscopy.

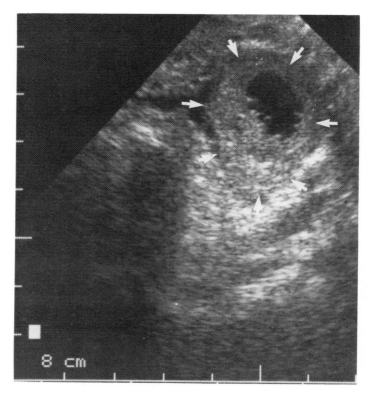

FIGURE 4.5 The wall of this slightly dilated and fluid-filled tube (outlined by arrows) is thickened. Clinical signs of an acute pelvic inflammatory disease were present.

The lumen of the tube is seen if it has been outlined by fluid or other contrasting material (eg, blood or a gestational sac). It is reasonable to suggest that if the lumen of the tube is brought into view and is distended, a pathological salpinx is present.

The contents of the tube may be a sonolucent, possibly serous (Figs 4.5–4.8), or more uniformly echogenic fluid such as a mucous or purulent fluid (Fig 4.9).

Blood clots may fill the tubal cavity, and after scans of several patients with ruptured tubal pregnancies, it would appear that blood clots in the tube present a complex and more difficult diagnostic task (Fig 8.6).

An unruptured *gestational sac,* with or without active embryonic heartbeats, is relatively easy to recognize by transvaginal sonography because of the natural fluid/tissue contrast created by the fluid-filled sac (Fig 8.4).

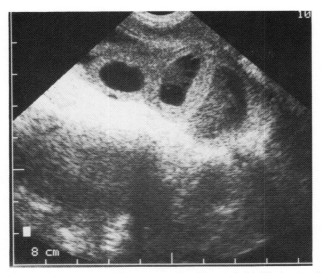

FIGURE 4.6 Cross section of three loops of a dilated, fluid-filled tube. Its walls are thickened. The patient was known to have occluded tubes and, at the time of the scan, had a tubal pregnancy in the contralateral tube.

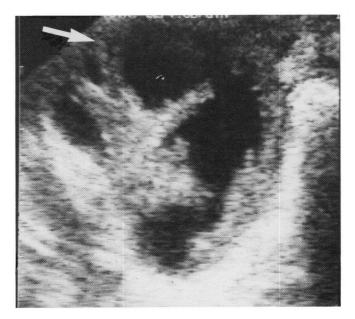

FIGURE 4.7 An occluded, dilated, fluid-filled sactosalpinx is evident. Some of the folds of the endosalpinx are still present. The distal end is marked with an arrow.

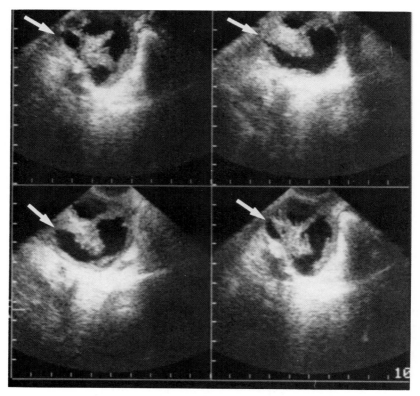

FIGURE 4.8 Serial cross sections of the tube shown in Figure 4.7. The proximal end is marked by arrows.

Mobility of the tube may be determined by attempting to move, displace, and even change the position of the tube (or the adjacent ovary) with a push–pull motion of the probe under direct observation on the scope. If no adhesions are present, a free sliding movement of the pelvic organs will be appreciated. This procedure is called the "sliding organs sign" and is described in Chapter 2. A chronically affected salpinx usually shows the same picture on repeated TVS examinations.

INFLAMMATORY PROCESSES OF THE TUBE

Two entities are of importance and therefore are mentioned:

1. Inflammatory processes of the tube are the hydrosalpinx or the pyosalpinx, dilated, fluid-filled, sometimes club-shaped structures (Figs 4.5–4.9).

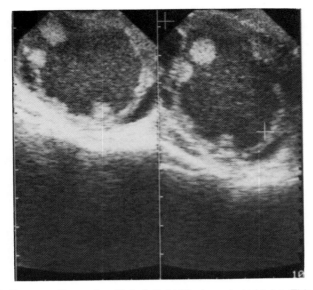

FIGURE 4.9 Cross sections of a dilated, fluid-filled, occluded tube. This patient was observed for ovulation induction in the in vitro fertilization program and had no complaints. The occluded right tube was diagnosed by salpingography. Note the thin wall with several thickened longitudinal folds of the endosalpinx.

2. Inflammatory processes of the tube and the ovary, namely the *tubo-ovarian abscess* (TOA), are usually adnexal conglomerates consisting of a dilated, fluid-filled tube in close proximity with an equally diseased, affected ovary.

The sonographic image of the TOA by the transvaginal probe is typical (Figs 4.10–4.12). A series of dilated, fluid-filled, round, thick-walled structures is apparent. Cross sections of the tube may show differences in size, but careful scanning in either plane will reveal the continuity of the tortuous lumen of the thick tube (Fig 4.11). The tube usually "embraces" the ovary, which loses its typical structure of stroma and follicles. Some of the ovarian follicles may still be recognized, thus enabling localization of the "ovarian part" of the TOA (Figs 4.10 and 4.11).

This tubo-ovarian conglomerate may be at its acute or its chronic stage. It also may appear as a result of recurrent flare-up in a patient with known previous pelvic inflammatory disease (PID). Spontaneous or elicited pelvic pain may be used to differentiate between acute and chronic cases of TOA.

An attempt may be made to bring this pelvic mass into the center of

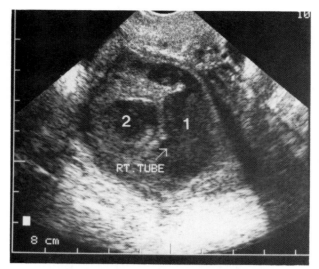

FIGURE 4.10 The tubo-ovarian complex is an entity easily recognized by TVS. The "tubal" part consists of the typical dilated tube (1). If the process is chronic, the wall of the tube is thin as in this picture. The "ovarian" part may show follicles or a cystic structure (2).

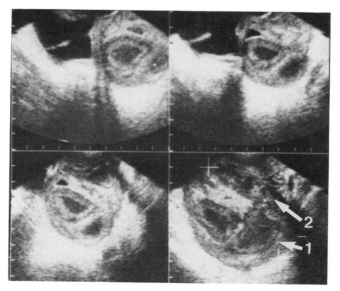

FIGURE 4.11 The acute phase of a tubo-ovarian abscess is shown. The tubal wall is thickened (1). The "ovarian portion," which is usually "embraced" by the dilated tube, is in the upper right of these sections (2). Pelvic fluid is evident on some of the images.

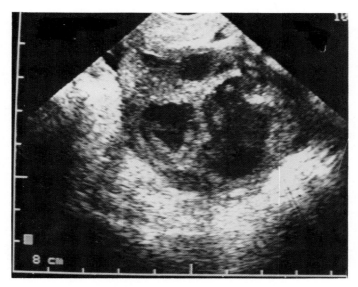

FIGURE 4.12 A left-side tubo-ovarian abscess in formation. The tube (1) and the ovary (2) are distended and difficult to recognize. This stage is one step away from pelvic abscess formation.

the scanning picture and then apply gentle pressure to evoke motion tenderness, which helps in the diagnosis.

With the above-mentioned sonographic picture one should look for the presence or absence of the "sliding organs sign." If no sliding of the *ovary* or the uterus is observed, either in relation to each other or to the pelvic wall, *adhesions* must be suspected.

An advanced case of TOA may show pelvic abscess formation consisting of larger, fluid-filled spaces without any possibility of recognizing the known anatomical structures of the tube or the ovary (Figs 4.12 and 4.13).

If tubo-ovarian pathology, or TOA, is diagnosed and emergency surgery is not considered or indicated, a series of follow-up examinations should be conducted to evaluate (a) the efficacy of conservative antibiotic treatment or (b) the appearance of a growing pelvic abscess that may need surgical intervention.

There has been speculation about the possibility of a transvaginal, ultrasound-guided fine-needle aspiration of pus for bacteriological workup, which may make early and adequate therapy possible.

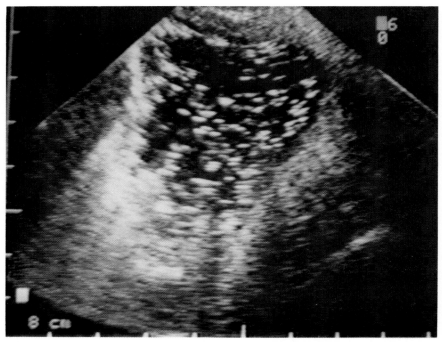

FIGURE 4.13 Image of a pelvic abscess. The tubal or ovarian structures cannot be demarcated. A large abscess resulting from rupture of a TOA was found at surgery.

TUBAL PREGNANCY

Tubal pregnancy is widely discussed in Chapter 8 and is mentioned here only because of its typical place in the list of tubal pathologies. Tubal pregnancy should always be suspected and, if possible, ruled out using multiple clinical, laboratory, and sonographic means.

MALIGNANCY OF THE TUBE

During the short time the authors have employed TVS there has been no opportunity to see this very rare entity. If clinical suspicion arises, it is felt that one should look for a thick-walled, stiff, fluid-filled structure much like the sactosalpinx. The severe mucorrhea inherent in and pathognomonic to its clinical picture will help in making the right diagnosis.

Differential diagnoses regarding the sonographic appearance of the salpinx require the following considerations:

1. A larger-than-average *ovarian follicle* possibly presenting as a dilated chronic hydrosalpinx. Its location in the ovary and adjacent to other smaller follicles, as well as its changing size through the menstrual cycle, makes the diagnosis simple.
2. A small *ovarian cyst,* which may mimic a thin-walled, distended hydrosalpinx. A carefully performed scan will invariably detect ovarian tissue as an integral part of this cystic ovary.
3. *Encapsulated fluid* in the pouch of Douglas presenting as hydrosalpinx or pyosalpinx. One should look for a contiguous tubal wall, which is not present in cases of peritoneal inclusion cysts.

In summary, the importance of TVS in tubal workup is one of its major strengths. It is the opinion of the authors, based on the outstanding ability of TVS to visualize a pathological or normal tube, that there has been a major breakthrough in pelvic sonography of the female patient.

Imaging of *tubal pathology* seems relatively simple to perform with the transvaginal probe, because most tubal lesions are connected with the presence of fluid (eg, blood or inflammatory fluid) around and in the Fallopian tubes. As discussed in previous chapters, this fluid serves as excellent "sonographic contrast material" for good imaging and diagnosis. On the other hand, imaging of a *normal salpinx* depends on the presence of the normally occurring free pelvic fluid. There is the possibility of selecting a midcycle day for the scan or placing the patient in a slightly reversed Trendelenburg position, but the obvious limitations preclude consistent imaging of the healthy tube.

Transvaginal sonography employing a higher-frequency transducer probe produces images with high resolution, opening realistic possibilities for a more reliable and clinically more meaningful diagnostic workup of the Fallopian tube.

REFERENCE

1. Davis FA, Gosink BB: Fluid in the female pelvis. Cyclic patterns. J Ultrasound Med 1986;5:75.

CHAPTER 5

The Ovary

Dan Beck, MD, Michael Deutsch, MD,
and Moshe Bronshtein, MD

Ovarian malignant neoplasms cause more deaths than any other female genital tract malignancy. Each year, 11,000 women in the United States die from this malignancy.

In spite of aggressive surgery, chemotherapy, and radiotherapy, no significant reduction in mortality has been achieved. More than two thirds of the patients are diagnosed when intra-abdominal spread is present (stage III), and only 9% to 28% of these will survive 5 years or more.[1,2]

More localized tumors (stages I and II) have a better 5-year survival: 50–70 and 42–52%, respectively.[1,3]

It is obvious that early detection is a primary concern for the clinician, but, unfortunately, early stages are usually asymptomatic. Increasing abdominal girth, discomfort, malaise, etc, are presenting symptoms associated with stage III disease.[1,2]

To improve survival of this ominous disease, different invasive and noninvasive modalities (ie, routine pelvic examination, cul-de-sac cytologic washing, markers in the serum, and different imaging modalities) have been suggested, but they have been used with inaccuracy and a low yield.[4] Further clinical aspects of ovarian cancer are beyond the scope of this book. The interested reader is referred to the relevant literature.[1-3]

In pre- and postmenopausal women, epithelial ovarian neoplasms account for at least 50% of benign ovarian tumors and 85% of primary malignant tumors. Malignant gonadal stromal and germ cell tumors are less frequent in this age group. In younger women, functional, epithelial, and benign germ cell cysts prevail.[1,3]

The serous cell carcinomas are the most common epithelial cancers.

59

These tend to be larger than 15 cm in more than 50% of the cases, and at the time of diagnosis *3.9% are less than 5 cm in diameter.*[1-3] The majority are composed of multilocular cysts with multiple papillary masses and solid nodules sometimes obliterating the cystic cavities. About 8% are solid adenocarcinomas without cystic elements. Benign serous cysts usually have no papillary masses on their inner surfaces. On the other hand, a smooth inner surface does not guarantee benignity.[2,5]

Tumor growth on the outer surface can be seen in almost half of the carcinomas, but this is also true in almost 10% of the benign lesions. Mucinous benign cysts tend to be larger, but size alone does not indicate malignancy.

The capsular surface is usually smooth, but firm mural nodules are common, and a few have intracystic papillae. Mucinous adenocarcinomas are usually cystic (approximately 76% multilocular and 24% unilocular[2]).

Other epithelial ovarian tumors also present a spectrum of cystic, solid, and papillary components.[2,5]

Germ cell and gonadal stromal tumors, benign and malignant, are usually solid.[2,5]

The dermoid cyst, which is a benign germ cell tumor, is usually characterized by multilocularity—sebum, fat, hair, and teeth, making its benign nature quite easy to evaluate macroscopically.[5]

Functional ovarian cysts are by definition nonneoplastic cysts (eg, follicular or lutein cysts). They are always monolocular with smooth inner and outer surfaces. These cysts, usually less than 5–6 cm in diameter, are common in young women. Observation of spontaneous regression is the proof of their benignity.[3,5]

It is obvious that the great diversity of ovarian tumors makes their macroscopic diagnosis in most cases inaccurate.

In certain early stages of ovarian tumors, histopathological evaluation is difficult and equivocal, depending on multiple sections of the tumor and on the skill of the pathologist.[2,5] It would therefore be an illusion to assume that sonography would be accurate in the histopathological diagnosis of ovarian tumors; however, the authors believe that one should review the relevant studies dealing with sonographic diagnosis of ovarian masses to place this diagnostic method in proper perspective.

ROLE OF TRANSABDOMINAL SONOGRAPHY IN OVARIAN DIAGNOSIS

Real-time sector transducer probes have been preferred for pelvic sonography over B-mode and linear transducer probes by most authors.[4,6-8] This preference has been due to the ability of the sector scanners to reach structures "hidden" by the symphysis or located deeper in the pelvis. Because of continuing improvement in transducer construction, as well as electronic image processing, certain characteristics of ovarian pathology may now be better defined. The characteristics to be sought are the smoothness of the inner cystic wall, inner and outer nodularity of cysts, septa, exact sequences of solid and cystic components, and inner content of ovarian cysts.

A short review of transabdominal sonography in pelvic imaging will illustrate its relative importance in diagnosing ovarian tumors.

Lawson, in a series of 251 pelvic masses, showed an accuracy of 91% in determining the existence, size, location, and consistency of pelvic lesions.[9] DeLand et al[10] predicted ovarian cancer by transabdominal sonography (TAS) in 13 of 14 patients. Only one of 38 ovarian tumors with a pure cystic pattern was malignant. In contrast, more than 70% of tumors with complex or solid patterns were malignant. Exact tumor size was predicted in about 90%.

Meire et al[11] showed a good correlation between sonography and pathology. In 23 women, all cystic masses smaller than 5 cm proved to be benign. In women in whom the cysts were unilocular but larger than 5 cm, 17 of 19 were benign, but in women in whom the cysts were larger and multilocular, 16 of 17 were malignant. Seven of 8 patients with thick septa and 15 of 18 with solid nodules had malignant ovarian tumors. Requard et al[12] tried to evaluate ascitic, peritoneal, omental, and lymph node spread of ovarian cancer and to characterize gross appearance of pelvic masses. Gross appearance was predicted accurately by sonography in 26 of 31 cases. The false negativity for predicting spread was high: 75% for lymph nodes, 80% for omental and peritoneal spread, and 16% for ascites. There were no false-positive cases.

Campbell et al[13] proposed sonographic criteria for diagnosis of ovarian neoplasia in menopausal women, in whom every palpable ovary is by definition suspected to be malignant. The sensitivity and specificity of their results were not established.

The use of sonography prior to second-look laparotomy, which is a well-established procedure,[1] was evaluated by Sonnendecker and Butterworth, who reported a high inaccuracy with this diagnostic tool.[14]

Wicks et al[15] showed that in clinically suspicious disease, sonography had 95% sensitivity, as opposed to 20% in unsuspected disease. Specificity was 92% and 100%, respectively.* Ovarian volume was suggested by Sample in 1977[20] to correlate with the endocrinological status of the pa-

---

* Sonographic characteristics of pelvic masses are described by several authors.[6,7,16,17] The most recent and comprehensive summary can be found in *Seminars in Ultrasound,* September 1983.[18,19]

tient. The problem was that the volume changes from puberty through pregnancy and postmenopause. Nomograms were compiled for ovarian size as a function of life cycle and as a function of the menstrual cycle itself.[21] This volume calculation depends heavily on exact ovarian measurements.

An enlarged ovary is not necessarily a pathological one, but ovarian tumors, or polycystic ovaries, are associated with an increase in ovarian size in the overwhelming majority of cases.

Since the long-term prognosis for patients with ovarian tumors and more specifically, for patients with ovarian carcinoma has been correlated with the extent of their resection, sonographic evaluation of tumor size may plan an important role in patient care. Despite all the technical achievements and the vast amount of literature on transabdominal ultrasonographic diagnosis of ovarian pathology, it seems appropriate to begin a discussion on this subject with quotes from O'Brient et al: "Sonography has changed the practice of obstetrics and has significantly affected gynecologic diagnosis" [highlighted by the editor], and "sonography was inferior to clinical examination" in the evaluation of the gynecologic patient.[22] Indeed, it "changed" obstetric diagnosis and management, but only "affected" gynecologic practice!

Similarly, Rifkin summarizes "where ultrasound stands today. . . . In summary: diagnostic ultrasound can now provide generally accurate differentiation of the normal and abnormal pelvis and an accurate picture of the female reproductive system. Unfortunately, sonographic results alone rarely permit exact tissue diagnosis."[23]

In short, transabdominal sonography, at this time, is able only to differentiate the normal from an abnormal pelvis. This falls short of the expectations of the gynecologist and the gyneco-oncologist.

ROLE OF TRANSVAGINAL SONOGRAPHY IN OVARIAN DIAGNOSIS

In this section, the role of transvaginal sonography in the evaluation of ovarian masses is discussed, but first it is important to mention the anatomical landmarks that help to locate the ovaries. They usually are situated laterally and slightly posteriorly to the uterus and often touch the internal iliac vein, but it is not unusual to detect at least one ovary in the cul-de-sac. Their "sonographic markers" are the follicles. The disappearance of the follicles, as well as their shrinkage, explains the difficulty in detecting ovaries with sonographic equipment in the postmenopausal years.

Ovarian imaging becomes easier if fluid is present in the pelvis. The volume may vary from several milliliters to full-blown ascites. Ovarian imaging by sonography correlates with the amount of pelvic fluid. The amount of naturally present fluid increases at mid-cycle[24]; thus, the potential for detecting the ovaries at this time is greater.

An additional way to enhance ovarian detection and examination with the transvaginal probe is for the examiner to place the other hand on the lower abdomen, to bring the adnexa closer to the tip of the vaginal probe. This maneuver is identical to the bimanual gynecological examination. It is important to note that some of the adjacent organs may mimic the ovaries or ovarian pathology; for instance, fluid-filled bowel, stool in the sigmoid or rectum, hydrosalpinx, ectopic pregnancy, and hematoma or fat tissue. An awareness of this possible pitfall during scanning or film reading is valuable.

After taking advantage of the outstanding resolution of the 6.5-MHz vaginal probe for egg retrieval in the in vitro fertilization program, as well as for the evaluation of very early intrauterine pregnancy and for detection of ectopic pregnancy, we turned to the process of learning the characteristics of the female pelvis, especially ovarian masses.

One hundred thirty patients with suspected pelvic masses of different size and consistency were referred for transvaginal sonography assessment. In 33 patients, final diagnosis was evaluated by the pathologist on the laparotomy specimen. The numbers were too small to determine the specificity and the sensitivity, and we could draw no conclusions based on extensive statistical analysis.

A few typical pictures representative of our ovarian workup are given here.

1. The *normal ovary* is relatively easy to locate and detect. In the reproductive years, it is disclosed by sonographic "markers"—the follicles or the corpus luteum (see also Chapter 9)—as well as by the clear sound interface created by the smooth surface and dense ovarian tissue (Fig 5.1). Because of its mobility the healthy, normal-sized ovary may change its location in the pelvis during transvaginal scanning. Normal amounts of pelvic fluid sometimes help outline the ovary (Fig 5.2).

   If abdominal or pelvic fluid (ascites or blood) is present, the ovary is easily found by TVS (Fig 5.3). The description of normal-appearing ovaries constitutes valuable sonographic information for the gynecologist and the gyneco-oncologist.

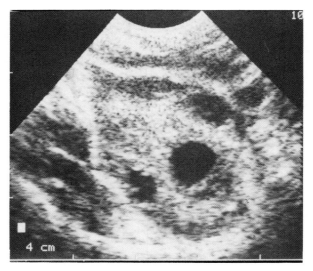

FIGURE 5.1 Transvaginal sonographic image of a normal ovary with three follicles—its sonographic markers.

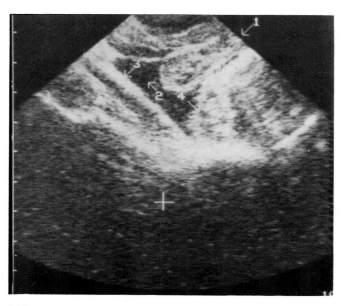

FIGURE 5.2 The normal right ovary (1) is outlined by normal amounts of fluid (2). The right hypogastric vein (3) marks the lateral wall of the pelvis.

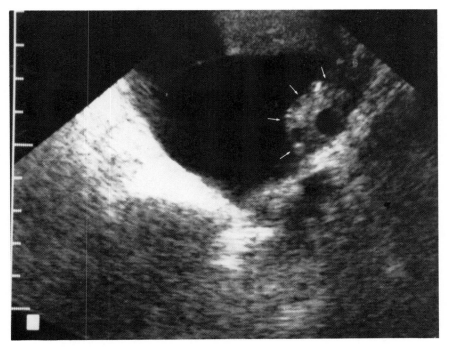

FIGURE 5.3 Ascitic fluid clearly outlines a normal ovary defined by several follicles (arrows).

2. The *polycystic ovary* has a typical sonographic appearance[25,26] and is recognized as a larger, spherical or almost spherical ovary with multiple small (less than 10 mm), immature follicles crowded along its surface (Fig 5.4). If the patient is hormonally stimulated, the image of the polycystic ovary is even more evident (Fig 5.5).

3. The *corpus luteum cyst* should also be mentioned here since it is a frequent finding and originates in the ovary. It is usually spherical and well delineated from its surroundings. Irregular echogenicity with bizarre formations in the cyst (fibrin-containing blood clots?) alternate with fluid phases (Fig 5.6). If followed by serial scanning, it decreases in size and the normal ovarian tissue is soon recognized in close proximity. The corpus luteum cyst may rupture, in which case sonographic diagnosis becomes extremely difficult; however, the free blood and blood clots are easily seen in the pelvis.

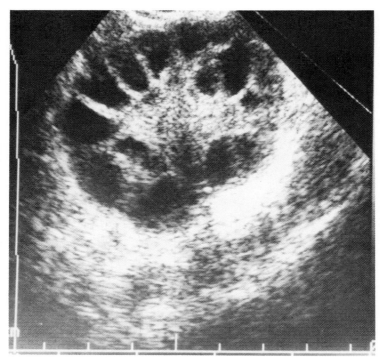

FIGURE 5.4 Small follicles are crowded at the surface of a spherical polycystic ovary.

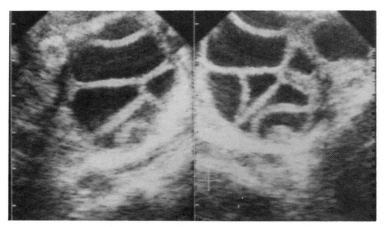

FIGURE 5.5 Image of a polycystic ovary after hormonal stimulation for enhancement of ovulation. Note that the enlarged polygonal follicles seem to be restricted from assuming a more rounded appearance by the typical thickened ovarian "capsular" structure inherent in this syndrome.

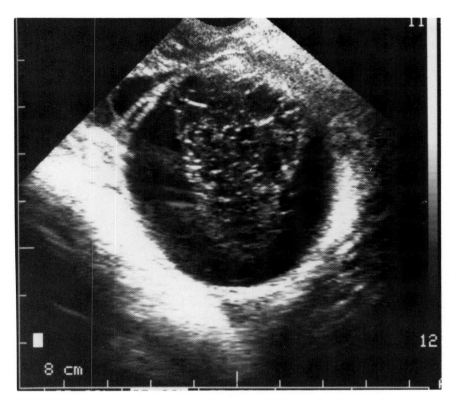

FIGURE 5.6 This corpus luteum shows an irregularly shaped and echogenic "cavernous" structure surrounded by a sonolucent area of fluid. Laparoscopy reinforced the sonographic diagnosis. The cavernous structure resembles the blood clot depicted in Figure 8.9.

4. *Functional (simple) cysts* (Figs 5.7 and 5.8) are always solitary cysts and are usually less than 6 cm in diameter. Transvaginal sonography is used to measure precisely the diameter of the cyst and follow its shrinkage. The cystic wall should be examined meticulously to exclude any nodule and/or papillary structures that are incompatible with functional cysts.

5. *Cysts with nodules or papillae* on the inner (Figs 5.9–5.12) or outer surface (Fig 5.13) may indicate true neoplastic cysts.[2] Differential diag-noses are benign epithelial cyst, cystadenocarcinoma (Figs 5.11 and

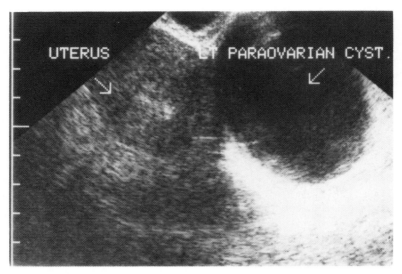

FIGURE 5.7 A 6.5 × 4.5 × 5.0-cm paraovarian cyst. A normal ovary was seen in another plane. Direct inspection and the pathological report confirmed the diagnosis suggested by TVS.

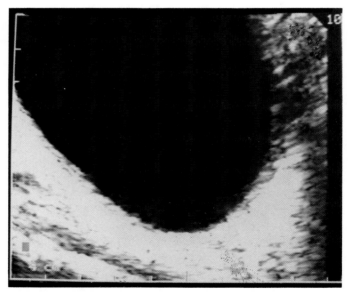

FIGURE 5.8 The smooth inner lining and the sonolucent contents of this 10 × 7 × 6-cm cyst suggest a benign appearance. No malignancy was detected by pathology.

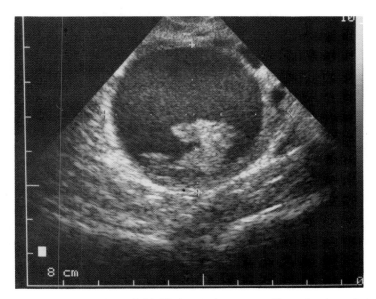

FIGURE 5.9 This 4.9 × 4.2-cm fluid-filled cyst shows a papillary structure. A dermoid cyst was reported by the pathologist. No malignant changes were detected in the papillary formation.

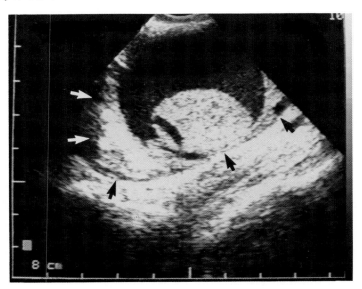

FIGURE 5.10 Another form of a protuberance in a cyst measuring 4.2 cm. Part of the ovarian border is outlined by arrows. The pathological report was dermoid cyst.

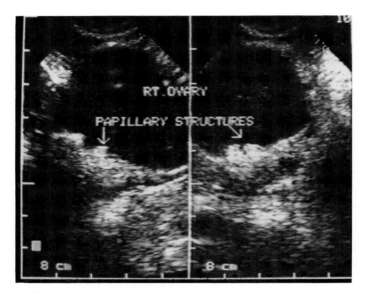

FIGURE 5.11 Papillary structures on the inner surface of a cyst. Adenocarcinoma was the pathological diagnosis.

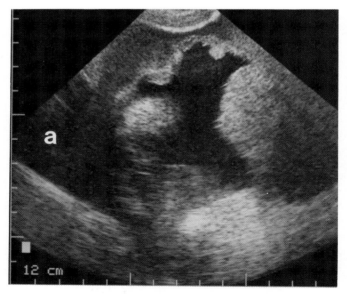

FIGURE 5.12 One of many partly cystic, partly solid tumors surrounded by ascites (a), showing nodular structures of various sizes. The pathological report was ovarian adenocarcinoma.

5.12), and dermoid cyst (Figs 5.9 and 5.10). If ascites are present as well, the probability of malignancy is higher (Figs 5.12 and 5.13). Nodularity or peritoneal implants may be detected in the presence of ascites (Fig 5.13).

6. *Multilocular cysts* are diagnosed easily by transvaginal sonography and suggest a diagnosis of epithelial cyst (benign or malignant) or dermoid cyst (Fig 5.14). As observed, their internal structure and septa show a variety of patterns.

7. *Dermoid cysts* are usually filled with a sebaceous substance that presents a typical sonographic pattern with the 6.5-MHz transducer. If filled with sebaceous fluid, these cysts tend to be spherical or ovoid in shape. The homogeneously echogenic contents of the cysts are obvious if scanned with a 6.5-MHz probe (Fig 5.15a), but they retain their sonographic properties even if a 5-MHz probe is used and pre- or postprocessing of the image is performed (Fig 5.15b). Their echogenicity is higher than that of clear fluid but much lower than that of a solid tumor (Fig 5.16). There is a similarity between the sonographic appearance of the sebaceous contents of a dermoid cyst and that of an endometrial (chocolate) cyst containing thick viscous blood. The dermoid cyst may contain hair, which, because of its high density, produces a typical acoustic shadow (Fig 5.17). The typical hairball may change its position within the cyst. This can easily be detected if the patient is tilted to both the left and the right during scanning, while the probe is still in place. In our small series of 13 dermoid cysts, one was multilocular (Fig 5.14c).

8. Because of a highly viscous blood filling, *endometrial (chocolate) cysts* (Figs 5.18 and 5.19) usually assume a spherical shape. They may also be molded by the available space, as well as by the pressure of adjacent organs (Fig 5.19b). These cysts may be part of the ovary (Fig 5.18), in which case the ovarian component is easily recognized. In other cases, the cyst is larger and the ovarian remnant is hard to find and recognize (Fig 5.19b). The homogeneous echogenicity of its contents resembles that of the dermoid cysts. The clinical picture helps clarify the sonographic picture in these cases.

9. *Solid ovarian tumors* appear as highly, but irregularly, echogenic masses (Fig 5.16). Sometimes, their texture resembles that of a uterine fibroid. These tumors should be recognized and described by shape, echogenicity, and special tissue characteristics, and measured in all three dimensions. The most common differential diagnosis is a pedun-

culated subserous uterine fibroid. Transvaginal sonography has the potential to differentiate between these two by (a) comparing the structure of the mass with that of the uterine muscle; (b) detecting a possible tissue "bridge" connecting the mass and the uterus; and (c) using the "sliding organs sign" (described in Chapter 2) to observe possible and extensive sliding of the adnexal mass over the uterus. In the case of a pedunculated uterine fibroid, the pelvic mass will slide over the uterine body, but detection of a normal ovary will help in establishing the diagnosis of uterine fibroid.

10. *Mixed tumors* show an alternating solid and cystic internal structure and histologically may be benign or malignant.

FIGURE 5.13 Four images of a 63-year-old patient diagnosed with stage III ovarian carcinoma. (**a**) Irregular tumors surrounded by ascites, and three nodular ¾-cm structures adhering to the pelvic floor. (**b**) More of the pelvic peritoneal seeding of the tumor outlined by the ascitic fluid. (**c**) The irregular outer surface of the echogenic (solid) tumor tissue amid pelvic fluid. (**d**) Atrophic uterus (u) surrounded by ascites. A small section of the ovarian tumor (arrow) is shown.

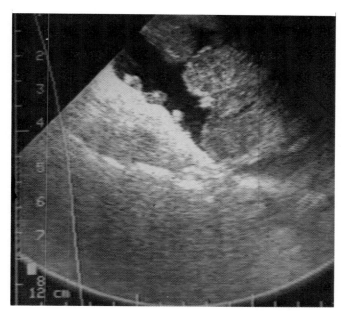

A

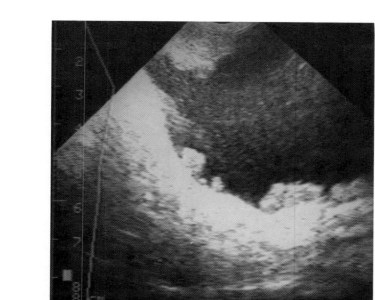

B

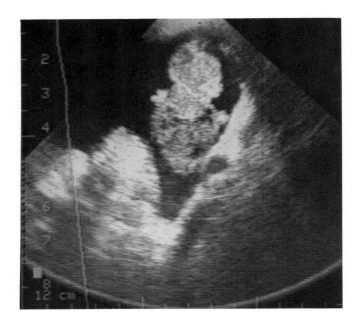

C

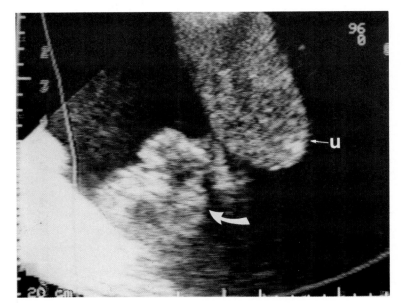

D

FIGURE 5.13 (*continued*)

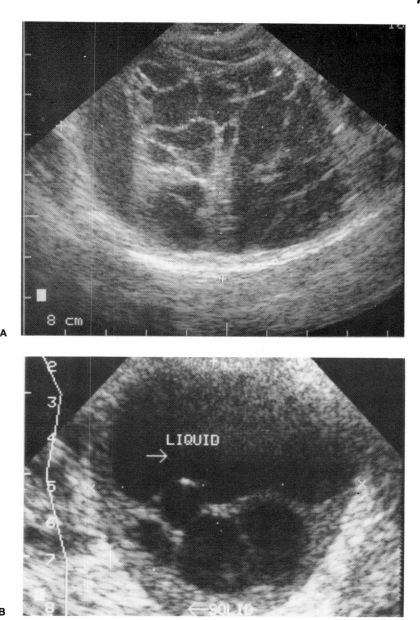

FIGURE 5.14 Three multilocular cysts show the intricate web of septa and echo-free fluid; all were subjected to pathological examination. (**a**) Benign cystadenoma. (**b**) Cystadenocarcinoma. (**c**) Dermoid cyst.

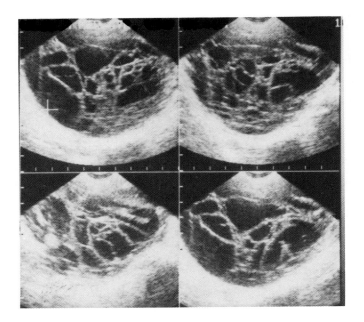

C

FIGURE 5.14 (*continued*)

FIGURE 5.15 (**a**) A 6 × 5.6-cm spherical cystic structure containing a uniformly echo-genic substance is depicted. (**b**) The same cyst imaged with a 5-MHz probe using different time-gain curves consistently shows uniform echogenicity higher than that of clear fluid. The cyst was an ovarian dermoid cyst containing sebaceous material.

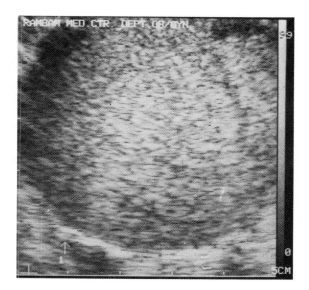

A

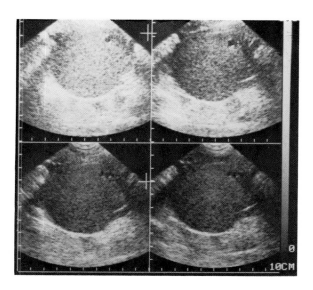

B

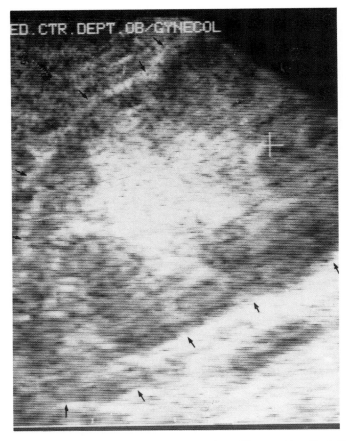

FIGURE 5.16 A solid, germinal 6 × 4.5-cm tumor in a 67-year-old patient. The highly echogenic "core" is surrounded by a lower echogenic peripheral region. No Graafian follicles can be seen at this age.

FIGURE 5.17 Two images of a right ovarian dermoid cyst. (**a**) Transabdominal image of a 9 × 8-cm tumor with a high echogenic round structure. (**b**) Transvaginal picture offering more detail: a uniformly low echogenic substance and a higher echogenic structure shifting its place when the patient is tilted from side to side, casting an acoustic shadow. At surgery, a "hairball" floating in sebaceous fluid was found.

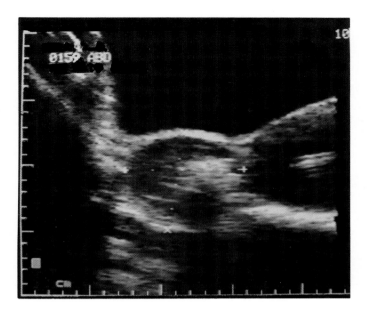

A

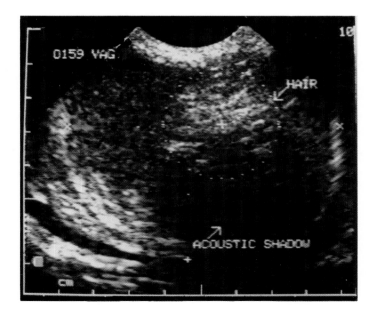

B

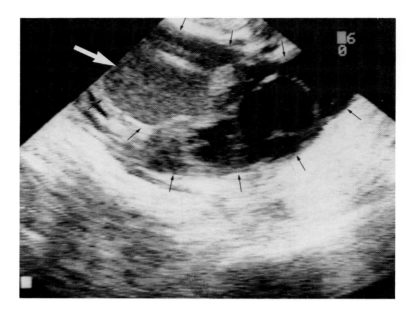

A

FIGURE 5.18 Serial sections (**a–c**) of an ovarian endometrioma. Small arrows outline the whole ovary containing the endometrial cyst (large arrow) and the normal ovarian tissue with several follicles (lower right side).

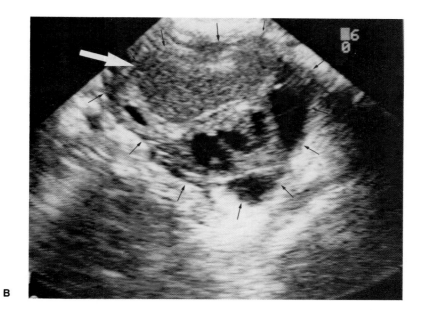

B

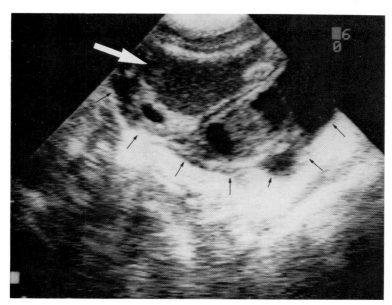

C

COMMENTS

In reviewing the literature, one clearly perceives that the sensitivity and specificity of the ultrasonic diagnosis of ovarian tumors have never been established in large series. Nor have good answers been found to the following questions: (a) What part does sonography play in the decision to operate? (b) Which patients might benefit most from sonography? (c) What are the clinical findings and conditions in which sonography would add considerable information?

Based on the literature and new insights, the authors suggest the following indications for performing a transvaginal scan, possibly with a high-frequency transducer probe:

1. To assess whether the pelvis is normal. This is especially important in evaluating obese and difficult-to-examine patients.
2. To further evaluate clinically found pathology. (Is it genital or does it belong to other viscera?
3. To characterize a lesion, even if only broad differential diagnosis will result from this scan.
4. To determine whether the sonographic appearance agrees with the clinical impression indicating surgery.
5. To determine with serial observations whether the mass is growing or regressing. These measurements are important in following a questionable functional ovarian cyst.[10]
6. To detect ascites that may be related to ovarian malignancy. Transvaginal sonography detects even minimal amounts of free abdominal fluid. If ascites are present, one should actively try to detect the ovaries. If in the presence of ascites *normal ovaries* are outlined (Figs 5.2 and 5.3), other possible causes for their presence should be sought.
7. To detect normal ovaries without ascites in the presence of a pelvic mass. This is valuable information for the gynecologist; therefore, a prolonged and meticulous search for the ovaries should be carried out even if pelvic masses are detected.

FIGURE 5.19 Large bilateral ovarian endometrioma scanned with a 5-MHz transvaginal probe. Note the uniformly echogenic thick blood contents (verified at operation) of the cysts. (**a**) The uterus (u) and the bilateral involvement are shown. (**b**) Part of the left ovary (arrows) is evident. TVS revealed that these cysts moved freely in the pelvis. No adhesions were found at surgery.

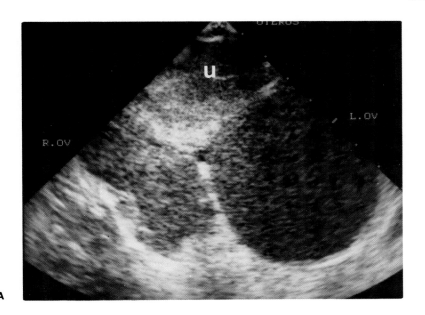

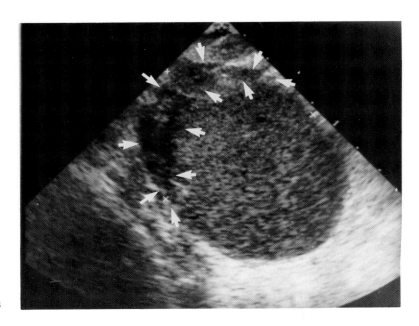

8. To evaluate the palpable ovary in postmenopausal woman. A noninvasive diagnostic modality seems to be more than desirable in these cases.[13]

9. To assess tumor response to chemotherapy (size, texture, place in the pelvis).

10. Possibly to avoid laparotomy in cases in which a suspicious pelvic lesion is found and biopsied under direct sonographic vision (the device used for biopsy is described in Chapter 9); however, sonography cannot replace second-look laparotomy.

11. To help evaluate the risk/benefit ratio for major surgical intervention in elderly and medically debilitated woman with pelvic masses.

12. To add information concerning the mobility of a pelvic mass ("sliding organs sign").

We should carefully examine the breakthrough in obstetrics introduced by sonography. In the modern management of pregnancy, sonography plays a major role. In evaluation of the female pelvis, sonography, in general, complements the physical examination of the patient. Transabdominal sonography with its inherent limitations should still be considered a basic and important part in the workup of the gynecological patient; however, we consider transvaginal sonography a more specific and more advanced diagnostic procedure for these patients. After a proper evaluation, TVS has the potential to close the gap between the heretofore clinically more valued obstetrical use of ultrasound and the relatively lower yield of transabdominal–pelvic sonography.

The authors believe that transvaginal sonography will soon become a routinely used diagnostic modality for the practicing gynecologist, as an adjunct to manual pelvic examination.

The use of transvaginal sonography, with its higher resolution, will inevitably lead to the detection of small-sized ovarian tumors.

Additional well-designed studies using transvaginal sonography as well as transabdominal sonography should be conducted as soon as feasible because of the possible superiority of the former method in the evaluation and early detection of ovarian pathology. This, in turn, will challenge gynecologists and oncologists to face and solve newly created gynecological problems, such as the very small ovarian tumor, which was "hidden from view" until now.

REFERENCES

1. Disaia P, Creasman W: Advanced epithelial ovarian cancer, in Clinical Gynecological Oncology, 2nd ed. St. Louis, Mo, CV Mosby Co, 1984, pp 286–360.
2. Hart W: Pathology of malignant and borderline epithelial tumors of ovary, in Coppleson M (ed): Gynecologic Oncology. London, Churchill Livingstone, 1981, pp 633–654.
3. Disaia P, Creasman W: The adnexal mass and early ovarian cancer, in Clinical Gynecologic Oncology, 2nd ed. St. Louis, Mo, CV Mosby Co, 1984, pp 254–285.
4. Smith L, Oi R: Detection of malignant ovarian neoplasms: A review of the literature. 1. Detection of the patient at risk; clinical, radiological and cytological detection. Obstet Gynecol Surv 1984;39:313–328.
5. Scully R: Atlas of Tumor Pathology. Tumors of the Ovary and Maldeveloped Gonads. Bethesda, Md, Armed Forces Institute of Pathology, 1979.
6. Garrett W: Ultrasound, in Coppleson M (ed): Gynecologic Oncology. London, Churchill Livingstone, 1981, pp 254–257.
7. Bernadino M, Dood G: Imaging of the pelvic contents in the female oncologic patient. Cancer 1981;48:504–510.
8. Nash C, Alberts D, Suciu T, et al: Comparison of B-mode ultrasonography and computed tomography in gynecologic cancer. Gynecol Oncol 1979;8:172–179.
9. Lawson T, Albarelli J: Diagnosis of gynecologic pelvic masses by gray scale ultrasonography: Analysis of specificity and accuracy. Am J Roentgenol 1977;128:1003–1006.
10. Deland M, Fried A, Van Nagell J, et al: Ultrasonography in the diagnosis of tumors of the ovary. Surg Gynecol J Obstet 1979;18:346–348.
11. Meire H, Farrant P, Gulta T: Distinction of benign from malignant ovarian cystology ultrasound. Br J Obstet Gynecol 1978;85:893–899.
12. Requard K, Mettler F, Wicks J: Preoperative sonography of malignant ovarian neoplasms. Am J Radiol 1981;137:79–82.
13. Campbell S, Goessens L, Goswamy R: Real time ultrasonography for determination of ovarian morphology and volume. Lancet 1980;1:425–426.
14. Sonnendecker E, Butterworth A: Comparison between ultrasound and histopathological evaluation in ovarian cancer patients with complete clinical remission. J Clin Ultrasound 1985;13:5–9.
15. Wicks J, Mettler F, Hilgus R, et al: Correlation of ultrasound and pathologic findings in patients with epithelial carcinoma of the ovary. J Clin Ultrasound 1984;12:397–402.
16. Quinn S, Erickson S, Black W: Cystic ovarian teratomas: The sonographic appearance of the dermoid plug. Radiology 1985;155(2):477–478.
17. Rosenberg E, Trought W: The ultrasonographic evaluation of large cystic masses. Am J Obstet Gynecol 1981;139:579–586.
18. Hall D: Sonographic appearance of the normal ovary, of polycystic ovary disease, and functional ovarian cysts. Semin Ultrasound 1983;4(1):149–165.
19. Williams A, Mettler F, Wicks J: Cystic and solid ovarian neoplasms. Semin Ultrasound 1983;4(1):166–183.
20. Sample W, Lippe B, Gyepes M: Gray-scale ultrasonography of the normal female pelvis. Radiology 1977;25:477–483.
21. Queenan J, O'Brien G, Baris L, et al: Ultrasonic scanning of ovaries to detect ovulation in women. Fertil Steril 1980;34:99–105.
22. O'Brien WF, Buck DR, Nash FD: Evaluation of sonography in the initial assessment of the gynecological patient. Am J Obstet Gynecol 1984;149:598–602.

23. Rifkin MD: Using ultrasound to diagnose gynecological malignancy. Contemp Obstet/ Gynecol 1984;23:200–205.
24. Davis FA, Gosink BB: Fluid in the female pelvis, cyclic patterns. J Ultrasound Med 1986;5:75–80.
25. Swanson M, Sauerbrei EE, Cooperberg PL: Medical implication of ultrasonically detected polycystic ovaries. J Clin Ultrasound 1981;9:219–222.
26. Parisi L, Tramonti M, Casciano S, et al: The role of ultrasound in the study of polycystic ovarian disease. J Clin Ultrasound 1982;10:167–172.

CHAPTER 6

Transvaginal Sonographic Assessment of Early Embryological Development

Zeev Blumenfeld, MD, Shraga Rottem, MD,
Sarit Elgali, and Ilan E. Timor-Tritsch, MD

To understand and appreciate the images produced by a 6.5-MHz transvaginal transducer probe, it is necessary to review several aspects of early embryological development. This short review is limited to a discussion of relevant highlights considered important in understanding some of the structures observed during scanning of early gestation.

CHRONOLOGY OF DEVELOPMENT
Preimplantation Period

In the rhesus monkey and in the human, the embryo reaches the uterus as a morula of about 16 cells still covered by the zona pellucida.[1] The early uterine morula in the human is about 0.1 to 0.2 mm in diameter,[1] a fact that must be appreciated if the events of implantation, ie, the attachment of the embryo to, and its embedment in, the endometrium, are to be understood. On the fourth or fifth day after ovulation, when the primate morula enters the uterine cavity, the endometrium is in the luteal phase and is approximately 5 mm thick. Its glands are actively secreting, and the walls are, therefore, covered by a film of mucus.[1] The morula is carried into the film of uterine secretion by the ciliary current from the uterine tube and lies free in it for the next 4 to 5 days. The mucosal surface is roughened by irregular depressions, most of which represent the openings of endometrial glands. These gland mouths may be wider than the diameter of the morula. The blastocyst may become lodged in or between these depressions as the first step in the attachment and implantation process. During this period, the morula loses its zona pellucida and develops into a spherical blastocyst, consisting of an outer layer of trophoblastic cells surrounding an inner fluid-filled blastocyst cavity and an inner cell mass. Also during this time, because of the absorption of fluid into its cavity from the uterine secretions, the blastocyst expands to a diameter of about 0.24 mm, but there is no increase in cytoplasmic substance. The oxygen and nutrient material required by the embryo at this very early stage are derived from the endometrial secretions. Until this point, no signs of pregnancy can be seen in any kind of sonographic examination.

Peri-implantation Period

The blastocyst has already attached and been partially implanted by 7–8 days after ovulation. The mode of early attachment of the human ovum is probably similar to that of the rhesus monkey, but the process commences at an earlier date. By the tenth or eleventh day postovulation, the human ovum becomes embedded in the endometrial stroma, partly because of the earlier attachment and partly because of the greater activity of the invading trophoblast. The stroma shows edema and congestion, which may result from the action of some substances produced by the implanting trophoblast and which may partly explain the degeneration of the uterine epithelium overlying this edematous stroma. Still, the edema and thickening of the endometrium observed on ultrasound examination are not yet diagnostic of pregnancy. This congested and edematous stroma provides nutritive material for the trophoblast, which now thickens rapidly at the region of contact where it differentiates into two layers: the original, inner, cellular *cytotrophoblast* or Langhans' layer, and the outer *syncytiotrophoblast* layer covering the cytotrophoblast and forming the layer of actual contact with the maternal tissues. The defect in the uterine epithelium caused by penetration of the ovum is gradually closed by a coagulum of fibrin and by proliferation of the adjacent epithelium. This method of embedment is called interstitial implantation, and at its completion the ovum lies in the superficial part of the stratum compactum, projecting slightly into the uterine lumen. After implantation of the blastocyst, the endometrium is called decidua and is divided into three topographically distinct portions depending on its relationship to the blastocyst: decidua capsularis, decidua basalis, and decidua parietalis (Figs 6.1a and 6.1b). The blastocyst normally implants in the endometrium of the uterine body, most frequently on its upper posterior wall. Because of this location, the transvaginal transducer probe is in closer proximity to the embryo than the transabdominal scanner.

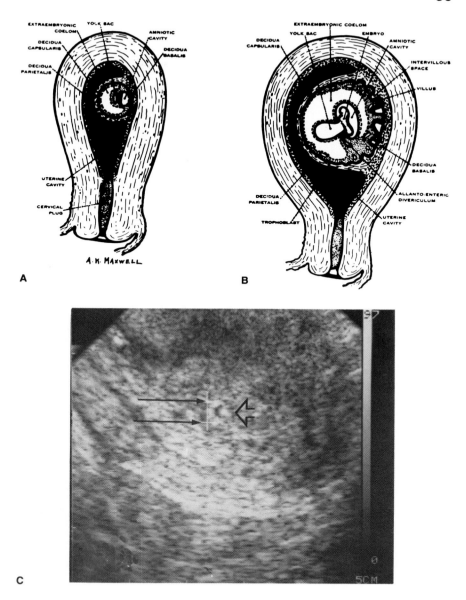

A

B

C

FIGURE 6.1 Diagrammatic representation of 5-week (**a**) and 6-week (**b**) embryos. Note the relationship among the decidua parietalis, decidua capsularis, and decidua basalis. (**c**) A normal 4-week 4-day intrauterine pregnancy. Only the gestational sac (open arrow) can be seen with TVS at this early stage. The gestational sac is only 4 mm in diameter (between long arrows).   (*continued*)

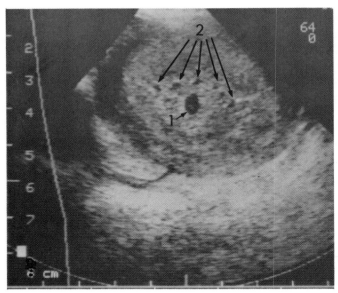

D

E

FIGURE 6.1 (*continued*) (**d**) Normal 5-week 0-day intrauterine pregnancy. The first structure that can be seen within the gestational sac is the yolk sac (1). Note the lacunar intervillous spaces (2) at this stage (as in Figs 6.1**b** and 6.2). (**e**) Normal 5-week 2-day pregnancy. Note the yolk sac within the gestational sac. (Figures 6.1**a** and 6.1**b** are reproduced from Human Embryology[1] by permission of The Macmillan Press Limited.)

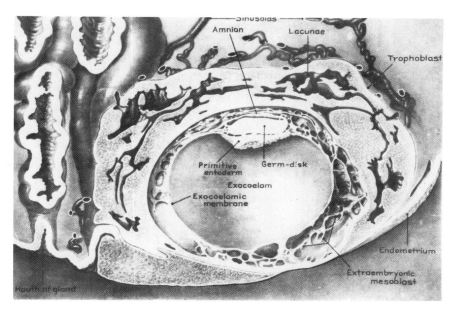

FIGURE 6.2 Day 11 of embryonic development (after ovulation). Note the primitive yolk sac, the extraembryonic mesoderm, and the lacunae at the depth of the implantation site of the gestational sac. (Reproduced by permission of The Macmillan Press Limited, from Human Embryology.[1])

The trophoblast is not uniformly developed over the surface of the implanted blastocyst, being thicker on its deep aspect (ie, toward the decidua basalis) than on its superficial aspect (decidua capsularis). This is probably due to the poorer supply of nutrients to the trophoblastic cells nearer the uterine lumen, and may be recognized on transvaginal sonography by the thicker trophoblast on the deep aspect of the gestational sac, the future placenta.

After the morula has become a blastocyst, a primitive yolk sac (Fig 6.2) lined by a single layer of trophoblastic cells forms. This layer of trophoblastic cells proliferates inward toward the primitive yolk sac (Fig 6.2), forming the extraembryonic mesoderm, and outward toward the uterine epithelium.[2,3] The primitive yolk sac decreases considerably in size. In the inner cell mass of the blastocyst, the amniotic cavity forms (Figs 6.1a and 6.1b). Within the extraembryonic mesoderm, another cavity—the extraembryonic coelom—forms (Fig 6.3), and this progressively surrounds the primitive yolk sac (Figs 6.3 and 6.4). The extraembryonic

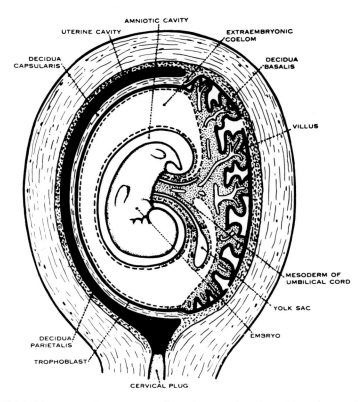

FIGURE 6.3 Diagrammatic representation of a 6-week embryo. Note the amniotic cavity surrounded by the extraembryonic coelom, and the intervillous spaces in the early placenta. (Reproduced by permission of The Macmillan Press Limited, from Human Embryology.[1])

coelom eventually surrounds the amniotic cavity, and, from that time, the remaining yolk sac is called the secondary yolk sac. The amniotic cavity and the secondary yolk sac are connected to the trophoblast by the connective stalk that prefigures the umbilical cord.

At about the fourth gestational week (since the last menstrual period [LMP]), the germinative layer, located between the amniotic cavity and the secondary yolk sac, progressively differentiates to produce the fetus (Fig 6.5). The outer aspect of the extraembryonic coelom is contained within the original trophoblastic layer, which proliferates on one side of the implantation to form the placenta and on the other side to form the

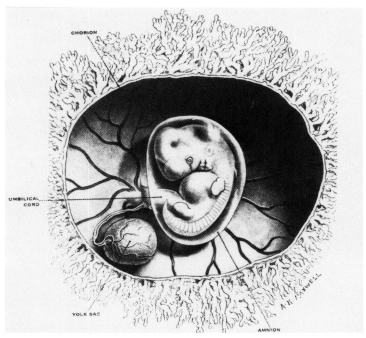

FIGURE 6.4 A 5½-week embryo. Note the relationship of the yolk sac and yolk stalk to the umbilical cord. Once the amniotic sac grows to encompass and obliterate the extraembryonic coelom, the yolk sac is incorporated into the umbilical cord and is only rudimentary. (Reproduced by permission of The Macmillan Press Limited, from Human Embryology.[1])

chorionic membrane. The portion of the chorionic membrane opposite the implantation adherent to the decidua capsularis separates the virtual uterine cavity from the extraembryonic coelom (Figs 6.1, 6.3, and 6.4). With the growth of the fetus and its amniotic cavity, the secondary yolk sac is squeezed by the amniotic cavity against the extraembryonic coelom. The yolk sac (Fig 6.4) now decreases in size and is connected by the vitelline duct through the connective stalk to the fetal abdomen. The anatomic features of the developing fetus, starting with the fetus and moving outward (Figs 6.1, 6.3, and 6.4), are the amniotic fluid, the amnion, the extraembryonic coelom, the decidua capsularis, the uterine cavity, the decidua parietalis, and the myometrium.[3]

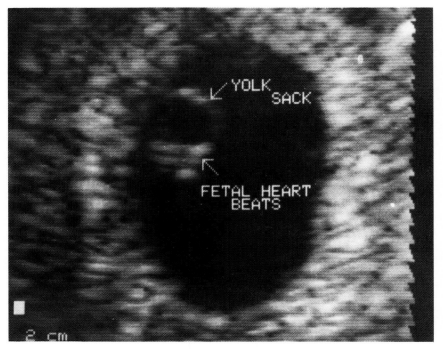

FIGURE 6.5 A 6-week 1-day intrauterine pregnancy. Note the yolk sac which at this early stage is larger than the embryo. The gestational sac measures 16 × 12 mm. At this early stage, fetal heartbeats can be detected by TVS at the place marked.

Development of the Fetal Circulation

During implantation, maternal blood comes into direct contact with the trophoblastic syncytium lining the lacunae.[1] This blood is a new source of nutrition for the embryo and its membranes. With this source of nutrition established only a fraction of a millimeter from it, the embryo itself rapidly differentiates. At 5 weeks after LMP, transvaginal sonography is able to detect and clearly show lacunar formations at one pole of the implanted gestation. These lacunar structures show distinct flow and, as seen in Figure 6.1**d,** they form a one-quarter to one-half circle around the gestational sac. At first the nutrients reach it by diffusion, but in the surprisingly short time of about 13 days after commencement of implantation (20-day-old embryo or 34 days from LMP), a simple circulatory system is formed in the embryo, chorion, yolk sac, and connective stalk. This precocious development of the embryonic heart and blood vessels is correlated with the rapid enlargement of the chorionic vesicle.[1] By the 21st day postimplantation, 5 weeks of gestational age (1.5 mm embryo), circulation from the embryo through the blood vessels is established and the fetal heart is pulsating. This, as said before, may be seen by the sixth week of gestation (from the LMP) only by transvaginal sonography. Thus the detection of fetal heartbeats by transvaginal sonography becomes possible within a week of its chronological development.

THE MATERIAL

The authors studied material gathered from approximately 215 pregnant patients and selected for this publication only those pregnancies that were carefully dated and whose images could be reproduced in other similarly well-dated gestations. For precise dating, the reliable first day of the last menstrual period was used as were basal body temperature measurements and hormonal assays. Several patients participated in the in vitro fertilization/embryo transfer (IVF/ET) program. For these patients, hormonal induction of ovulation was followed by sonography. Gestational ages given here were calculated in weeks and days from the first day of the LMP. If hormonal follicular stimulation and ovulation induction were used, the gestational age was calculated starting with the day of ovulation as day 14 of the cycle (or the last day of the second week).

In a small pilot group, assays of serum human chorionic gonadotropin, β subunit (β-HCG), were performed daily starting on day 28 of the cycle. The levels obtained were correlated with transabdominal and transvaginal sonographic detection of the early gestational sac. At the time of the ultrasound examination, β-HCG levels were not known to the physicians involved in the scan.

WHAT DOES TRANSVAGINAL SONOGRAPHY SEE IN EARLY PREGNANCY?
Fifth Week

The gestational sac can usually be detected at 4 weeks 1–4 days from the LMP (or 15–18 days after ovulation). The average level of serum β-HCG at this gestational age is 400–800 mIU/mL. At this time the gestational sac measures 4–5 mm and is usually detected within the "shining" endometrium. In one of these carefully dated pregnancies, the gestational sac was detected at 4 weeks 1 day and measured 4.2 mm. The serum β-HCG was found to be 820 mIU/mL on the same day. The lowest serum β-HCG level

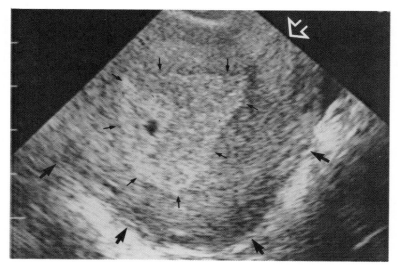

A

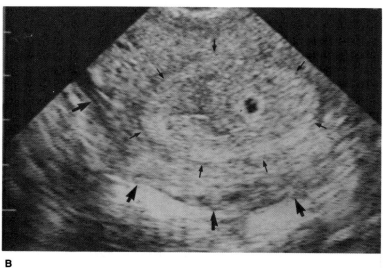

B

FIGURE 6.6 (**a**) Transvaginal sonographic picture of a 4-week 1-day intrauterine pregnancy. The serum β-HCG level was 420 mIU. In this longitudinal (vertical) section the cervix points to the right (open arrow). The endometrium is highlighted by small arrows, and the posterior aspect of the uterus, by large arrows. (**b**) Transverse section of the same uterus.

at which a gestational sac was detected was 420 mIU/mL; the gestational age was 4 weeks 1 day (Fig 6.6).

By the end of the fifth week, transvaginal sonography detected all intrauterine gestation in patients with well-documented dates. On the average, the transabdominal 3.5-MHz sector transducer probe detected the gestational sac for the first time about 1 week after the 6.5-MHz vaginal probe produced its first image of the same patient.

Sixth Week

Although diagnosis of pregnancy at this gestational age is possible, but difficult, by transabdominal ultrasound,[3] it becomes *feasible* and *relatively easy with transvaginal sonography* (Figs 6.1c and 6.6). An important characteristic of the early gestational sac is the double line, differentiating it from other intrauterine elements, such as uterine bleeding or the decidual reaction of a pseudogestational sac, described in ectopic pregnancies. These have a single echogenic rim and may suggest an erroneous diagnosis of intrauterine pregnancy.

The origin of the double contour or double ring at this gestational age has been attributed to the rapidly proliferating inner cytotrophoblast and outer syncytiotrophoblast. One or two weeks later, the hyperplastic endometrium is "invaded" by the trophoblast, thus creating the decidua basalis and chorion frondosum on one side and the decidua capsularis and parietalis (or vera) on the other side. All of these contribute to the later sonographic appearance of the previously described echo-dense ring around the true intrauterine gestational sac.

Two structures deserve to be mentioned:

1. The yolk sac becomes evident at 5 weeks 0 days and fills about one third of the cross section of the gestational sac. At this time it measures 4 mm (Figs 6.1d and 6.1e). Its cross section in a normal pregnancy is always a circle because of its spherical shape. Transabdominal sonography will consistently detect the yolk sac from 6 weeks onward (Figs 6.5 and 6.7). The potential clinical importance of the yolk sac is discussed in Chapter 7 in conjunction with the missed abortion.

2. Lacunar structures of 2–3 mm are appreciated by transvaginal sonography on one side of the gestational sac (Fig 6.1d). They are located along a curved line forming about one fourth of a circle. Flow was clearly seen in these structures when a high frame rate was employed. The authors believe that these vascular elements are the forerunners of the maternal placental circulation. They are described in classic textbooks of embryology.[1,2]

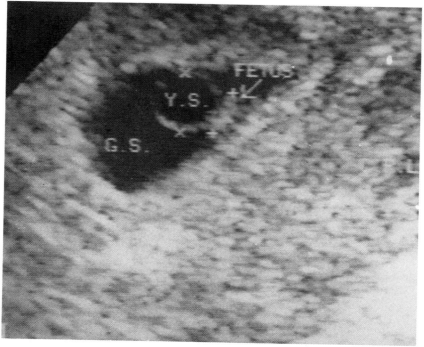

FIGURE 6.7 In this 7-week 2-day pregnancy, the gestational sac (G.S.), yolk sac (Y.S.), and fetal pole (fetus) are shown. The fetal pole measures 5 mm. Heartbeats are evident on real-time scanning.

Seventh Week

A 15-mm cystic structure representing the gestational sac (Fig 6.5) is outlined with great precision by transvaginal sonography. The main "landmark" now is an echogenic fetal pole consisting of the 2- to 3-mm embryo adjacent to a cystic yolk sac. One should remember that the yolk sac is an extraembryonic structure. The amniotic membrane is the partition between the two (see Figs 6.4 and 6.8). Fetal heartbeats are seen from 6 menstrual weeks onward. On several occasions in well-dated pregnancies, we were able to locate fetal heartbeats at 5 weeks 5 days from the LMP. The double contour is now much more evident. The thickness of the trophoblast should be one fifth to one third of the diameter of the gestational sac, and must be included in the measurement of the sac.[3] Throughout the sixth and seventh weeks, the fetal pole becomes more evident but measurements are still not feasible for dating purposes. It

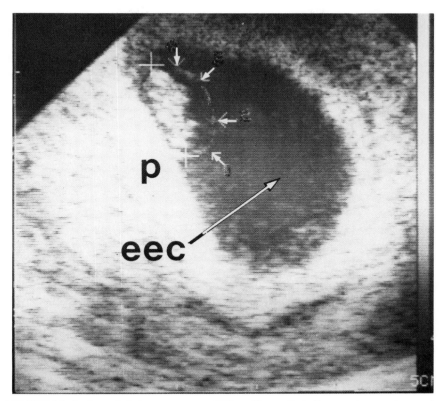

FIGURE 6.8 An 8-week 0-day pregnancy. CRL = 12 mm. Note the membranes (arrows), the placental site (p), and the large extraembryonic coelom (eec). The yolk sac is normal but visible in a different plane.

would appear that tables and graphs of crown–rump lengths compiled from data obtained by transabdominal sonography may not be as accurate as believed, because they were obtained by the transabdominal approach with a transducer of relatively low resolution; thus, part of the yolk sac may have been included in the measurements. This confusion, or rather imprecision, is reflected in the recent literature.

Eighth Week

The gestational sac has increased in size to 22 mm, and the fetus can be perceived clearly by the vaginal route. The trophoblastic rim is only one-fifth to one-fourth the thickness of the gestational sac. From the seventh week onward, measurements of the gestational sac are less informative but the crown–rump length (CRL) measurements become meaningful. Because of the high resolution, a clear outline of the fetal pole enables a precise CRL measurement at this very early stage of the pregnancy. The membranes are starting to appear by TVS.

Ninth Week

The placenta becomes more demarcated and its relationship to the uterine cavity may be extrapolated (Fig 6.8). At this stage the embryonic structure is represented by distinct parts of the fetal body—the head, trunk, and limbs. The size of the fetal head surpasses the diameter of the yolk sac and it becomes a distinct anatomical structure. It appears to be filled with fluid, but no differentiation to the left and right ventricular systems is yet visible (Fig 6.9a). The choroid plexus could not be detected at the beginning of this week of gestation. Normal growth can be estimated by the crown–rump length, which is easily measured at this age. The limb buds can be detected and the fetus can be seen moving freely within the amniotic cavity. The coccygeal region protrudes at this age and appears more prominent than the lower limb buds (Fig 6.9b). Close to the end of week 9 the choroid plexus can be seen on some of the images (Fig 6.10b). The amnion expands more and more at the expense of the extraembryonic coelom; flow is first seen in the tiny umbilical cord (Figs 6.10a and 6.10b).

Tenth Week

During this week the yolk sac slightly diminishes in size, starts to thicken, and is "pushed" aside by the continuously enlarging amniotic sac (Figs

---

FIGURE 6.9 (a) At 8 weeks 2 days, one single ventricle is visible in the head (1). The limb buds are prominent. (b) The lower part of the same fetus is magnified. The lower limb buds are marked by open arrows. The sacrococcygeal region (white arrow) is still prominent at this gestational age.

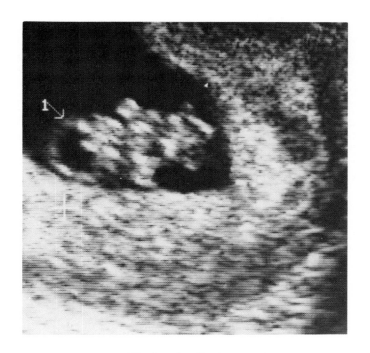

A

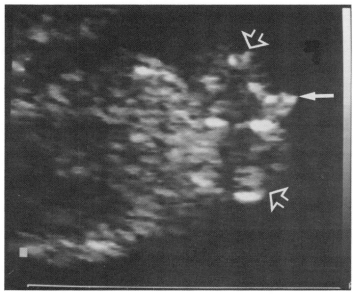

B

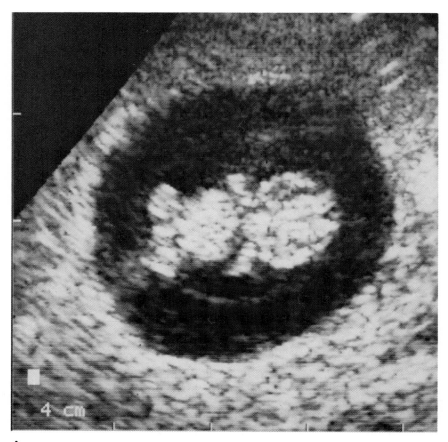

A

FIGURE 6.10 An 8-week 4-day normal fetus is shown. (**a**) Frontal section showing well-outlined head, trunk, and limb buds. CRL = 19 mm. (**b**) Longitudinal anteroposterior section showing the head with ventricle and choroid plexus, yolk sac (open arrow), and cord (double arrows) surrounded by the amnion (arrows).

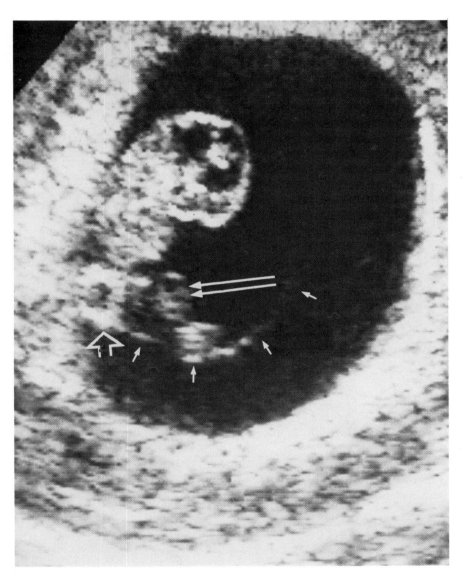

B

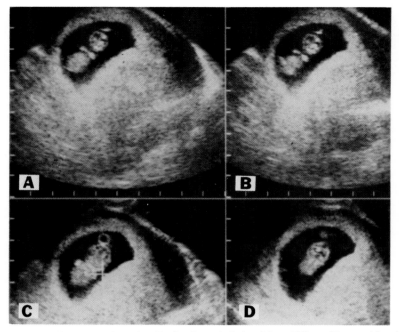

FIGURE 6.11 Serial sections (**a–d**) of a 9-week 2-day fetus. CRL = 25 mm; biparietal diameter = 9 mm. The amnion and the yolk sac are visible above the head.

6.11–6.13). This process involving the yolk sac continues into the tenth week at which time it is almost absorbed and incorporated into the umbilical cord.

The left and right lateral ventricular systems in the fetal head are now obvious and fill almost the entire volume of the skull. The highly echogenic choroid plexus is easily seen in both lateral ventricles (Fig 6.12).

Fetal movement is detected in all live fetuses at 10 weeks.

Tenth to Thirteenth Week

By the end of the first trimester the decidua capsularis adheres to the decidua parietalis. Thus the virtual uterine cavity (the extraembryonic coelom) is obliterated, and the "double contour" attributed to a normal intrauterine pregnancy in the earlier stages is no longer seen. At these gestational ages, precise measurements of fetal structures can be made; however, most available tables correlating these measurements with ges-

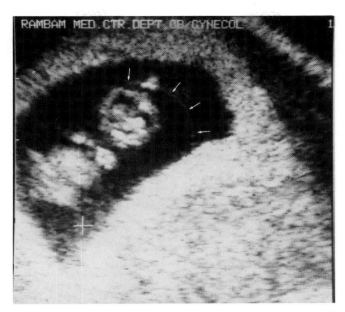

FIGURE 6.12 Enlarged image of Figure 6.11**b.** The ventricles and the partition into two hemispheres are visible. The left and the right choroid plexus are well delineated in the ventricles. Above the head a small segment of the yolk sac and the thin amnion are imaged (small arrows). The extraembryonic coelom (eec) is still extant at this age.

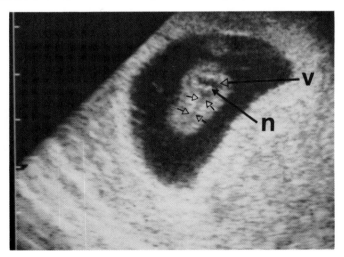

FIGURE 6.13 Enlarged image of Figure 6.11**d.** This coronal section of the fetal body crosses the fetal head and the spinal canal (pairs of small arrows); n = two minute protuberances into the ventricle (v), which may represent some of the midbrain nuclei.

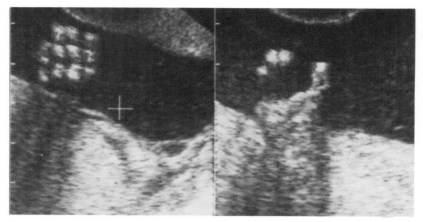

FIGURE 6.14 Hand of a 12-week 4-day fetus. The first scanning plane (**a**) depicts fingers 2–5; another plane (**b**) reveals the thumb.

tational age were based upon data generated by the transabdominal scanning route. Therefore, their "lower end" may not agree with those generated by the transvaginal probe.

From 12 weeks onward, the fetal hand (Fig 6.14) and foot can be examined for possible malformations. A significant number of chromosomal or other malformations are associated with those of the limbs and the digits.

The Cervix in Pregnancy

At this point it is important to discuss examination of the cervix during pregnancy. The two most important aspects of this examination are evaluation of dilation and the possible diagnosis of placental localization relative to the internal cervical os.

An example of a successful cervical scan during the first trimester is shown in Figure 3.2. In this picture an uneffaced, closed cervix can be appreciated 10 weeks into the pregnancy.

Evaluation of placental/cervical relationships in cases of spotting or slight vaginal bleeding during the first and second trimesters is easily done if indicated. A placenta previa is visualized in Figure 3.3 at 18 weeks. These aspects of evaluating the cervix in pregnancy are discussed in Chapter 3.

COMMENTS

The high resolution of the 6.5-MHz probe makes possible a closer look at the early pregnancy through more detailed imaging of different embryonic structures. This property of the higher-frequency transducer can be compared to the use of a high-power microscope to increase picture resolution. An important observation was made: almost every anatomical structure of early pregnancy was detected earlier by transvaginal than by transabdominal sonography. A closer look was taken at a selected group of 15 patients with well-documented and dated pregnancies. The performance of the generally used 3.5-MHz linear or sector scanner and the time of first detection of certain embryonic structures, as opposed to the 6.5-MHz transvaginal probe, were reviewed. The transvaginal probe detects the same embryological structures 1 week earlier, on the average, than the generally used, customary transabdominal probe. A more detailed list of the various structures examined is given in Table 6.1.

Transvaginal sonography has limitations in scanning late second-trimester as well as third-trimester fetuses. One limitation, obviously, is the advancing gestational age leading to a rapidly increasing volume of amniotic fluid and a fast growing fetus. Starting from the first days of the second trimester, the fetus literally outgrows the 2- to 7-cm "effective" focal zone of the 6.5-MHz transducer probe. A 5.0-MHz transvaginal probe can extend the focal range to about 10 cm at the expense of its resolution; therefore, its transvaginal use would no longer present an advantage. However, in the second trimester, because of an increase in

TABLE 6.1 Detection Times for Embryological Structures

Embryonic/Fetal Structure	Gestational Age at Detection	
	TVS	TAS
Gestational sac	4 wk 1–3 d	5 wk
Yolk sac	5 wk	6–7 wk
Fetal heartbeats	5 wk 6 d	6 wk 4–7 d
Limb buds	8 wk	9 wk
Head	8 wk	9 wk
Ventricles	8 wk 2–4 d	11 wk
Choroid plexus	9 wk	11–12 wk
Hand, fingers	12 wk	17–20 wk

Abbreviations: TVS, transvaginal sonography; TAS, transabdominal sonography.

amniotic fluid production, fetal presentation and position change more often. Thus, there is good reason to believe that the body part, or organ of interest, will potentially come within reach of the vaginal probe. If the resolution of a 6.5-MHz probe is needed to image a second-trimester or early third-trimester fetus, one or several attempts should be made with a reasonable expectation of success. The benefits of external maneuvering of the fetus into the desired position can also be considered against the low risk of this procedure.

Transvaginal evaluation of the cervix and placental location at times of vaginal bleeding may raise some controversy and, therefore, merit comment. We advise transabdominal sonography as the first step in the workup of second- and third-trimester vaginal bleeding. If for any reason (eg, unsatisfactory scanning, patient obesity) this examination does not lead to the expected sonographic diagnosis, TVS should be considered. As previously described (Chapter 3), the examination of the cervix starts and becomes optimal when the tip of the probe is still 3–5 cm away from physical contact with it. If a low-lying placenta or a dilating cervix is detected, the probe should be removed at once. Continuous documentation by tape-recording should be done.

In conclusion, transvaginal sonography detects various anatomical structures of the early pregnancy approximately 1 week earlier than the widely employed transabdominal scanning. We predict that this new method will be useful in the diagnosis of early and possibly second-trimester gestation as well as in learning more about early fetal anatomy and physiology. Careful judgment should precede the use of the vaginal transducer probe in cases of second- or third-trimester vaginal bleeding.

REFERENCES

1. Hamilton WJ, Boyd JD, Mossman HW: The implantation of the blastocyst and the development of the fetal membranes, placenta and decidua, in Human Embryology. Cambridge, W Heffer & Sons Ltd, 1945, pp 49–76.
2. Rock J, Hertig AT: Some aspects of early human development. Am J Obstet Gynecol 1942;44:973–983.
3. Jeanty P, Romero R: What does early gestation look like? in Jeanty P, Romero R (eds): Obstetrical Ultrasound. New York, McGraw–Hill, 1984, pp 34–40.

CHAPTER 7

Pathology of the Early Intrauterine Pregnancy

Ilan E. Timor-Tritsch, MD, Shraga Rottem, MD, and Zeev Blumenfeld, MD

In the previous chapter the role of transvaginal sonography in diagnosing the normal intrauterine pregnancy was described; the present chapter is closely related to the previous one and is, in many aspects, based on it.

Despite the fact that nonviable gestations ultimately undergo abortion, the uterus may not expel the products of conception for weeks. Thus, it is of some importance to identify correctly those gestations that are nonviable before complications occur. Among the complications may be prolonged uterine bleeding, septic abortion, and, of equal importance, psychological upset of the patient and her family.

About one quarter of pregnant women have uterine bleeding during the first trimester. It is believed that more than one half of these abort spontaneously.[1] Hormonal assays alone—one of the two main tools for evaluating the pregnancy—lack the ability to correctly determine all potentially nonviable gestations. The second tool is ultrasound. Pathological appearance of the gestational sac was once considered to be reliable evidence of an abnormal gestation.[2,3] Transabdominal sonography could correctly identify 53% of abnormal gestational sacs,[3] and transabdominal ultrasound, in conjunction with radioimmunoassay of human chorionic gonadotropin, β subunits (β-HCG), was found by Nyberg et al[4] to be useful in the diagnosis of early intrauterine pregnancy. The same author extended these studies to the pathological early pregnancy and reported on the successful use of simultaneous β-HCG level measurements and gestational sac size in the identification of abnormal gestations.[5] Previous studies reported that a gestational sac should be detected by transabdominal sonography when the β-HCG level is equal to or exceeds 6,500 mIU/

109

mL. This level of β-HCG was called the "discriminatory zone."[6] This "discriminatory zone" was recently updated by Nyberg et al.[4] They consistently demonstrated a normal gestational sac when the β-HCG level was greater than 1,800 mIU/mL. As they applied this cutoff level of β-HCG to ultrasound findings, a discrepancy was discovered between the sonographic finding and the expected β-HCG level: only 36% of abnormal pregnancies were detected by the hormonal assay. When gestational sac size was used in comparison with the β-HCG level, 65% of the abnormal gestations were detected.[5] Nyberg et al consider transabdominal ultrasound a reliable method of gestational sac assessment, but add that it "requires an experienced sonographer for correct interpretation."

The following are some of the morphological characteristics of an abnormal gestation detected by the *transabdominal method:*

1. A small-for-date gestational sac. This requires knowledge of accurate menstrual dates, which often are not known.[7]
2. The presence or absence of fetal heart motion by the end of the seventh menstrual week. Good dating of the pregnancy is crucial for this.[7–9]
3. The appearance of the gestational sac of irregular or even bizarre shape, an unnaturally large sac that lacks an embryo, the absence of the double decidual reaction ("double sac sign").[2,11]
4. An anembryonic pregnancy, which may result from an early embryo death or an embryo that never developed.[2,9,11]

Nyberg et al[3] further refined the morphological description of the abnormal gestational sac, which is considered as such if the following conditions apply:

1. It is larger than 24 mm without an embryo.
2. It has a distorted shape.
3. It has a thin choriodecidual reaction that measures 2 mm or less and no yolk sac is present.
4. The choriodecidual echoes are of low amplitude.
5. An irregular contour is seen.
6. The typical double gestational sac is lacking and the sac is greater than 10 mm.
7. The sac is in a very low position within the lower uterine segment.

Detection of one of the first three criteria by transabdominal sonography was associated with 100% specificity as well as a positive predictive value in diagnosing an abnormal pregnancy. Because of the ability of these sonographic signs to define missed abortion, they are considered "major criteria."

The remaining criteria are considered "minor criteria" because they are more subjective in their interpretation as well as somewhat less specific in diagnosing an abnormal gestation. Several of these "minor criteria" combined to raise the positive predictive accuracy to 100%. This high level of accuracy is needed when the decision is made to evacuate the uterus in the case of an abnormal gestation.

Following the first reports of the sonographic detection and description of the yolk sac,[12] several communications have pointed out its potential value in the diagnosis of a normal or abnormal gestation.[13–15] By transabdominal sonography the human yolk sac is viewed from the seventh week onward. At 10 weeks of menstrual age it starts to shrink, and by the eleventh week it is incorporated into the umbilical cord[12,15] (see Chapter 6). It should also be remembered that the yolk sac and the yolk stalk are extra-amniotic structures (see Figs 6.1, 6.3, and 6.4).

If the yolk sac is seen but no fetal pole is evident, the diagnosis of missed abortion should be made.[14] These criteria as well as a small-to-date and free-floating yolk sac were suggested by Hurwitz to be the "yolk sac sign."[15]

One should always emphasize that an abnormal-appearing gestation may develop normally. This seems to be the generally accepted clinical opinion. Therefore, caution must be exercised, and it is advisable to give the suspected threatened abortion the benefit of the doubt when there is a normal-appearing or mildly atypical gestational sac. The patient should be reexamined in 1 week.[3]

The aim of sonography in the diagnosis of possible pathology during early pregnancy is twofold: First is the reliable, early, and expeditious detection of a missed abortion to enable emptying of the uterus. This will shorten uterine bleeding and psychological upset of the patient. Similarly, it will reduce the rate of first-trimester complications. Second, if the pregnancy is normal, it will reassure both the patient and her obstetrician simultaneously.

Because of its higher resolution and unobstructed view in obese patients, transvaginal sonography should present certain advantages in the diagnostic algorithm of pathology in early pregnancy. From Chapter 6, it is clear that the basic embryological structures of the early gestation are seen about 1 week earlier with TVS than with transabdominal scanning. The prerequisite of accurate pregnancy dating must once again be stressed. In Chapter 6, we described the sonographic images of the early abnormal pregnancy as seen with the 6.5-MHz transvaginal transducer probe.

TRANSVAGINAL SONOGRAPHIC MORPHOLOGY OF THE ABNORMAL GESTATION

The following sonographic signs were considered by the authors as being consistent with an abnormal gestation. They may appear alone or in any combination and may involve (1) the uterus with its decidual reaction, (2) the gestational sac and its membranes, (3) the fetal pole itself, and finally (4) the hydatiform mole.

Uterus and Decidua

1. *Irregular appearance* of the normal echogenic decidual double ring with unclear lacunar structures (Fig 7.1).
2. *Partial or complete disappearance* of the echogenic double ring, the echogenicity of which approaches the lower echogenicity of the uterine muscles (Figs 7.1–7.3).
3. *Partial or complete detachment* of the decidua by fluid-filled spaces. Our speculation is that this fluid may indeed be blood (Fig 7.4).
4. *Complete disappearance of the products of conception* following spontaneous expulsion (Fig 7.3). This is usually confirmed by a previous positive pregnancy test as well as a previous ultrasound examination showing a clear gestational sac.

FIGURE 7.1 This 10-week intrauterine gestation (**a,b**) shows some of the characteristics of an abnormal pregnancy: the sac itself is small (23 × 16 × 15 mm) and irregular; a small yolk sac (1), an irregularly echogenic decidual ring, unclear lacunar structures, and a small, amorphous fetal pole (2) are also observed.

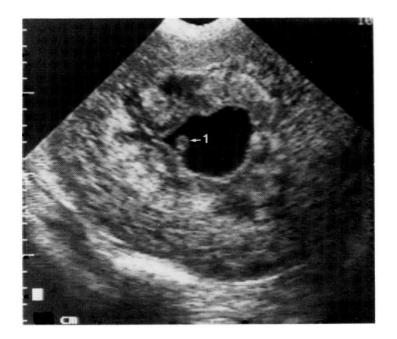

A

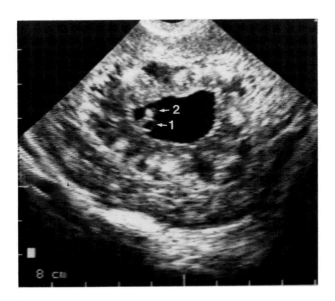

B

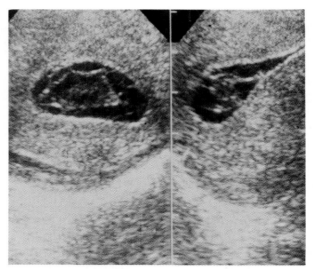

FIGURE 7.2 A 9-week pregnancy showing a "blurred" decidual ring, shrunken amniotic membranes, and an undefined, amorphous fetal pole. The left side is a cross section, the right side a longitudinal section, of the uterus.

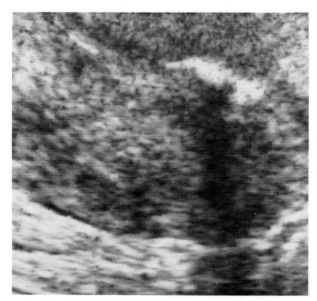

FIGURE 7.3 Transvaginal scan of an almost complete spontaneous abortion. Longitudinal section of the uterus showing the echogenic structures (blood clots?) along the cavity line. The cervix faces the upper left corner. Several days before, fetal heartbeats had been observed in a normal-appearing gestational sac.

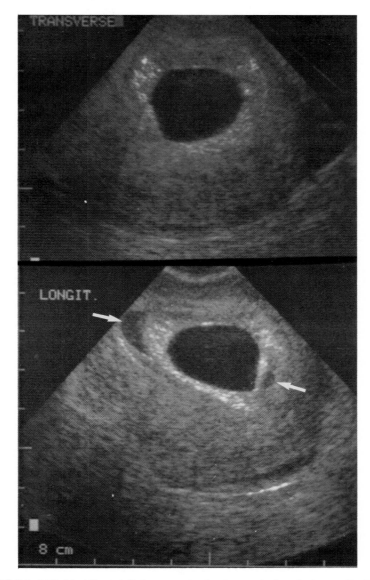

FIGURE 7.4 A blighted 8-week 5-day ovum is clearly seen in the uterine cavity. The sac is empty and measures 22 × 18 × 23 mm on the longitudinal section. Note the partial detachment of the decidual ring (arrows). The meaning of the strongly echogenic areas in the decidual ring is unknown.

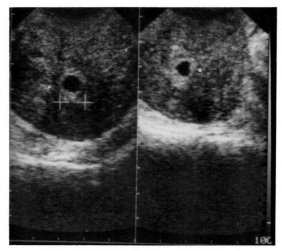

FIGURE 7.5 Vaginal spotting was the presenting symptom in this 6-week 3-day pregnant patient. The sac was 10 mm in diameter and was devoid of a yolk sac and a fetal pole. The decidual reaction seemed to be less echogenic than usual. Two cross sections are on the left; the longitudinal section is on the right.

Gestational Sac and Membranes

1. *Discrepancy between sac size and dates* (Fig 7.5). At 8 weeks menstrual age the sac size is about 25 mm. Different tables are available for use.

2. *An empty sac* 20 mm or larger is highly suggestive of an abnormal gestation (Fig 7.4).

3. *Irregularly shaped sac,* usually flat (Fig 7.6) or polygonal in shape (Figs 7.7 and 7.8).

4. *Detached membranes* (Figs 7.9 and 7.10). Multiple scans performed in successive sections and planes are necessary to make this observation (Figs 7.8 and 7.10).

5. *Irregular and shrunken amniotic membranes* (Figs 7.2 and 7.8), which may be completely detached from any supporting decidual tissue.

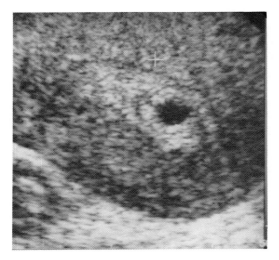

FIGURE 7.5 (*continued*)

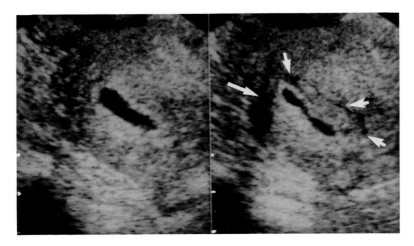

FIGURE 7.6 This flat gestational sac was found in a 7-week pregnancy. The "double-ring" sign can hardly be recognized, the sac is empty, and there is some detachment of the decidua (arrows).

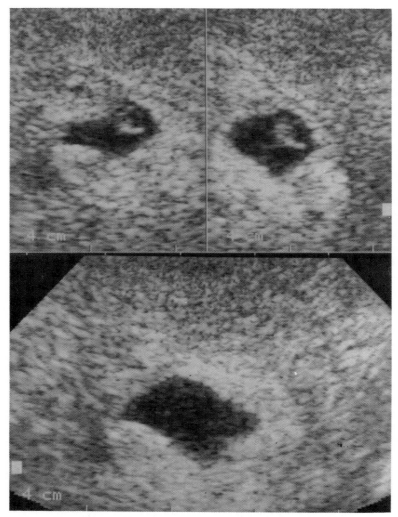

FIGURE 7.7 Characteristic features of a missed abortion detected with TVS: crumpled and shrunken gestational sac, rectangular sac, deformed or flattened yolk sac. No heartbeats were seen at 11 weeks.

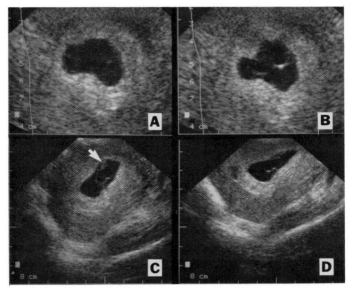

FIGURE 7.8 Four serial sections (**a–d**) of an 8-week abnormal pregnancy. (**a,b**) Cross sections showing fragments of membranes and the fetal pole. (**c,d**) Flat gestational sac; detached and shrunken membranes; small ill-defined, fragmented yolk sac (arrow); and poorly defined decidual ring.

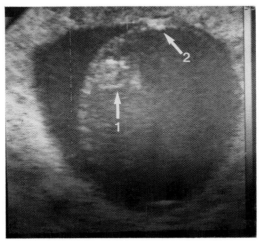

FIGURE 7.9 Completely detached spherical gestational sac in an 11-week 2-day pregnancy. No fetal heartbeats were detected during previous scans. Prominent signs of an abnormal gestation in this image are amorphous fetal pole (1) and small highly echogenic remnant of the yolk sac (2).

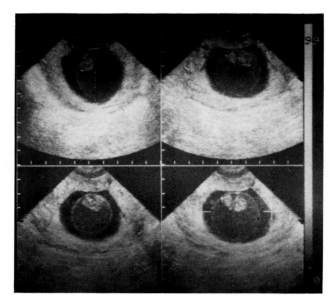

FIGURE 7.10 Four serial sections of the pathological pregnancy shown in Figure 7.9 are presented to demonstrate complete detachment of the amniotic sac floating freely in the gestational sac (measuring 5 cm). The amorphous irregularly echogenic fetal pole is obvious.

Fetal Pole and Yolk Sac

1. *Fetal pole.* The fetus itself may undergo *degenerative changes.* The transvaginal sonographic signs are an amorphous, irregularly echogenic, irregularly shaped tissue mass with no fetal heartbeats (Figs 7.1, 7.9, and 7.10).

2. *No visible fetal heartbeats* after 6½ weeks menstrual age. This has to be supported by accurate dating of the pregnancy or by previous, documented heart motion.

3. *The pathology of the yolk sac:*

   a. *Nonexistent yolk sac* (Figs 7.4 and 7.5), usually diagnosed along with an anembryonic gestation.

   b. *Smaller-than-4 mm yolk sac* (Figs 7.1, 7.8, and 7.9).

   c. *Irregularly shaped and irregularly echogenic yolk sac* (Figs 7.7 and 7.8c).

  d. *Fragmented yolk sac* (Fig 7.8c).

  e. *Freely floating yolk sac,* which may be observed on the real-time scan or at subsequent scans comparing images taken at the same plane or orientation.

Hydatiform Mole

The sonographic picture of the hydatiform mole is typical and is easily diagnosed by the transabdominal approach. The transvaginal approach should be used in obese patients or in patients in which the image obtained by transabdominal sonography is inconclusive. The sonographic picture obtained by transvaginal sonography shows a multitude of different-sized sonolucent structures with high fidelity (Fig 7.11); thus, a reliable diagnosis of hydatiform mole or molar degeneration can be made.

  Understanding the normal development of embryonic and fetal structures, as detected by transvaginal sonography, enables early recognition of blighted ova and missed abortions. Although the classical definition of "missed abortion" includes an 8-week interval between the chronological age and the uterine size, the term is more commonly used to define lack of

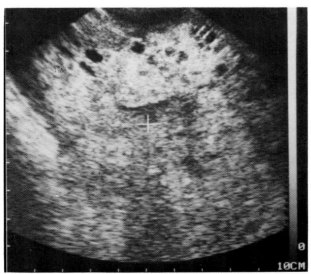

FIGURE 7.11 Hydatiform mole. The transvaginal image is typical, showing a large number of sonolucent round structures of various sizes.

normal development of the intrauterine pregnancy even before an 8-week lag between the size and menstrual age. According to the "classical" definitions, in cases of "*blighted ova*" the gestational sac remains "empty." No fetal pole nor yolk sac can be seen, as opposed to the sonographic picture of "*missed abortion*" showing several or most of the listed sonographic characteristics.

The diagnosis of "blighted ovum" or "anembryonic gestation" was initially made and suggested by transabdominal sonography. If early serial scans are performed with the higher-resolution 6.5-MHz transvaginal transducer probe, more precise observations may be made, leading to a change in our basic diagnostic approach regarding the abnormal pregnancy. For instance, we may learn that the blighted ovum is just another step in the natural process of an abnormal gestation.

Sonographic examination is the most appropriate laboratory tool in diagnosing any first-trimester pregnancy disturbance. If no definite answer as to the life of the embryo is obtained when transabdominal ultrasound examination is performed, one should use transvaginal sonography. In the pathology of pregnancy the diagnostic process is closely linked to a precise dating of the pregnancy itself. In the first trimester, exact dating is even more important since fundamental changes detected by transvaginal sonography appear every week starting from the fourth postmenstrual week. Knowledge of the exact dating will enable the clinician to determine the normal or abnormal progress of a very early pregnancy based on serial TVS and its findings. The reverse of this is also true: if the pregnancy proceeds normally but the gestational age is unknown or not certain, one may be able to "date" the pregnancy according to the known chronological appearance of the gestational sac, fetal pole without and with heartbeats, etc.

We assume that widespread introduction of transvaginal sonography will enable the construction of more meaningful and precise tables of gestational sac size that will correlate better with gestational age and with serum β-HCG levels. In their "pioneer work," Kadar et al[6] described a discriminatory zone: first detection of the gestational sac at serum β-HCG levels equaling at least 6500 mIU/mL using the transabdominal–transvesical route. In applying transvaginal sonography, this *discriminatory zone* has now been adjusted to a much lower level—500 or 800 mIU/mL—to reflect the high resolution of the 6.5-MHz transducer crystal used in this technique. This level is even lower than that proposed by Nyberg et al.[4]

Because of its high resolution, transvaginal sonography detects the basic embryological "landmarks" about 1 week earlier than transabdominal scanning (Table 6.1).

If, according to earlier work with transabdominal sonography, ultrasound alone was able to detect 53% of abnormal gestations,[3] we may speculate that the use of transvaginal sonography will increase the sensitivity and the specificity as well as the positive predictive value of detecting early embryonic pathology, thus enabling a more reliable diagnosis to be made *earlier.*

Finally, it is clear that transvaginal sonography opens new possibilities for morphological, physiological, and pathophysiological studies concerning early embryonic development. Basic embryological structures are detected 1 week earlier, on the average, by transvaginal sonography than by transabdominal sonography. Once basic, descriptive works are completed, clinical application will undoubtedly improve early embryonic diagnosis and therapy.

REFERENCES

1. Fantel AG, Shepard TH: Basic aspects of early (first trimester) abortion, in Iffy L, Kaminetzky HA (eds): Principles and Practice of Obstetrics and Perinatology. New York, John Wiley & Sons, 1981, vol 1, pp 553–563.
2. Donald I, Morley P, Barnette E: The diagnosis of blighted ovum by sonar. Br J Obstet Gynecol 1972;79:304–310.
3. Nyberg DA, Laing FC, Filly RA: Threatened abortion: Sonographic distinction of normal and abnormal gestational sacs. Radiology 1986;158:397–400.
4. Nyberg DA, Filly RA, Mahoney BS, et al: Early gestation: Correlation of HCG levels and sonographic identification. Am J Roentgenol 1985;144:951–954.
5. Nyberg DA, Filly RA, Duarte-Filho DL, et al: Abnormal pregnancy: Early diagnosis by VS and serum chorionic gonadotropin levels. Radiology 1986;158:393–396.
6. Kadar N, DeVore G, Romero R: Discriminatory HCG zone: Its use in sonographic evaluation for ectopic pregnancy. Obstet Gynecol 1981;58:156–161.
7. Anderson SG: Management of threatened abortion with real-time sonography. Obstet Gynecol 1980;55:259–264.
8. Hertz JB: Diagnostic procedures in threatened abortion. Obstet Gynecol 1984;64:223–229.
9. Robinson HP: The diagnosis of early pregnancy failure by sonar. Br J Obstet Gynaecol 1975;82:849–857.
10. Ericksen PS, Philipsen T: Prognosis of threatened abortion evaluated by hormone assays and ultrasound scanning. Obstet Gynecol 1980;55:435–438.
11. Jouppila P, Herva T: Study of blighted ovum by ultrasonic and histopathologic methods. Obstet Gynecol 1986;55:574–578.
12. Mantoni M, Pedersen JF: Ultrasound visualization of the human yolk sac. J Clin Ultrasound 1979;7:759–762.
13. Sauerbrei E, Cooperberg PL, Poland BF: Ultrasound demonstration of the normal fetal yolk sac. J Clin Ultrasound 1980;8:217–220.
14. Bernard KG, Cooperberg PL: Sonographic differentiation between blighted ovum and early viable pregnancy. Am J Roentgenol 1985;144:597–601.
15. Hurwitz RS: Yolk sac sign: Sonographic appearance of the fetal yolk sac in missed abortion. J Ultrasound Methods 1986;5:435–438.

CHAPTER 8

Think Ectopic

Shraga Rottem, MD,
and Ilan E. Timor-Tritsch, MD

EPIDEMIOLOGY

Reports indicate that during the last 15 years, there has been a marked increase in ectopic pregnancies throughout the world. In Sivin and Cooper's study[1] of 35,496 American women, the rate of ectopic pregnancy (EP) almost doubled between 1965 and 1976. Rubin et al[2] described an increase in rate from 4.5 to 9.4 per 1,000 reported pregnancies. In Sweden, the rate of EP increased from 5.8 to 11.1 per 1,000 conceptions in 15 years,[3] and in Great Britain, the rate per 1,000 live births and therapeutic abortions increased from 3.2 to 4.3.

Ectopic pregnancy accounts for a significant rate of maternal death (26% of all maternal deaths in the United States), a fetal wastage of nearly 100%, and a high incidence of maternal morbidity.[4]

In 1980, a 3-week delay in making the correct diagnosis was reported in 14.4% of cases.[5] We believe it is possible to shorten this diagnostic delay time with the use of higher-resolution ultrasound equipment together with the β-HCG assay which is available most hours of the day. Nevertheless, the diagnostic and therapeutic problems of ectopic pregnancy are far from being solved.

The basic reason for the increase in the rate of EP is the fact that more adolescent girls are sexually active; with this comes sexually transmitted disease as well as pregnancy. The microorganisms causing ectopic pregnancy are usually the chlamydiae and *Neisseria gonorrhoeae,* but other microbes may be implicated in the resulting salpingitis as well. Therefore, it becomes increasingly important to consider ectopic preg-

125

nancy in the differential diagnosis of a teenager presenting with abdominal pain and irregular vaginal bleeding.

The chance of recurrence after one EP varies from 5 to 20%. Some women with a previous EP develop problems of infertility and never deliver a living child. According to Curran's projection, by the year 2000 at least 10% of all females of reproductive age will become involuntarily sterile as a result of the sequelae of pelvic inflammatory disease; more than 3% will experience an ectopic pregnancy.[6]

Ongoing improvements and the results of in vitro fertilization programs should not diminish efforts to improve prevention, diagnosis, and treatment of ectopic pregnancy.

NONINVASIVE DIAGNOSIS OF ECTOPIC PREGNANCY

The noninvasive diagnostic "triangle" of the "think ectopic" concept consists of clinical presentation, laboratory tests, and ultrasonographic scanning, detailed as follows.

Clinical Presentation

It is well known that the patient suspected of having an ectopic gestation presents with the triad of pain, abnormal vaginal bleeding, and pelvic mass; however, these signs are nonspecific and frequently misleading. Only 45% of a group of 245 patients suspected of ectopic pregnancy had the above-mentioned "classic triad."[7] Even in accordance with modern trends, it is not superfluous to mention the statement of Howard Kelly: "If one is confronted with a pelvic condition which follows no rules and conforms to no standards one should think of ectopic pregnancy, particularly if she has any menstrual irregularity and has incurred the risk of pregnancy." Other clinical signs may be amenorrhea, which is usually followed by irregular vaginal bleeding; shoulder pain; an enlarged soft uterus; vertigo; fainting; and shock. Symptoms need not always be present and are insufficiently precise to enable the diagnosis of an early ectopic pregnancy before rupture and intraperitoneal bleeding and their devastating consequences.

Pregnancy Tests

These tests are based on the determination of human chorionic gonadotropin (HCG). The amount of HCG doubles every 2 days, reaching a peak of 100 IU/mL at a gestational age of 6 weeks.[8] The first commercially available tests for HCG were immunological tests performed on blood or urine samples. The frequent false-positive and false-negative results, as well as the fact that they become positive about a week after a missed period, limited their effectiveness.[8] The HCG molecule cross-reacts with other hormones and medications and shows a false-positive result in hematuria, in proteinuria, and, to add to the confusion, in tubo-ovarian abscess.[9] The cross-reactivity of HCG in ectopic pregnancy and in cases of tubo-ovarian abscesses was particularly worrisome because of the clinical closeness of the two entities.

The false-negative results of the HCG assay in EP probably result from the low titer of hormone produced by the relatively small amount of trophoblastic tissue.[10]

Because of the limited value of the immunological HCG assay in differentiating between a normal intrauterine pregnancy and a very early EP (low sensitivity and specificity), clinicians sought more accurate ways of determining low titers of HCG. Introduction of the radioimmunoassay made possible measurement of levels of 0.1 IU.[11] The test is specific for the β chain of the hormone and, therefore, does not cross-react with other hormones or chemical compounds.

The levels of β-HCG are closely correlated to the normally developing gestation, and because a negative result excluded pregnancy with 100% confidence,[10] this pregnancy test came into widespread use. Modifications of the laboratory procedure significantly reduced the time in which a result could be obtained by the clinician.[12] As a result of these advances, determination of the β-subunit of HCG became one of the cornerstones of correct diagnosis of ectopic pregnancy.[7,13,14]

Sonography

The third noninvasive clinical tool in the workup of the patient with suspected faulty implantation of the embryo is sonography. A vast amount of literature deals with various aspects of the sonographic diagnosis of ectopic gestation. The diagnosis was usually made by viewing an empty but slightly enlarged uterus along with an adnexal mass and, sometimes, fluid in the cul-de-sac.[15] Over the years it became obvious that the "classic" sonographic findings of EP were not always present[15,16]; despite notable technical advances made in the last decade, transabdominal–transvesical sonography did not provide the expected solutions to the diagnostic problem presented by ectopic gestation. A significant contribution to the earliest possible diagnosis of ectopic gestation, using transabdominal ultrasound in conjunction with determination of β-HCG levels, was made by Kadar et al in 1981.[17] They introduced the "discriminatory zone" of 6,500 mIU/mL at which a normal intrauterine gestational sac should be detected. Nyberg et al, using more advanced sonographic equipment, reduced this "discriminatory zone" to 1,800 mIU/mL or greater, levels at which they were first able to detect a normal intrauterine pregnancy.[18]

Unfortunately, transabdominal (transvesical) sonography (TAS) reaches diagnostic accuracy only by the seventh postmenstrual week of gestation. The false-positive rate of diagnosis ranges between 3 and 30% (mean 16%); the false-negative rate is lower: 2–35% (mean 5%).[19] Since diagnosis of ectopic pregnancy is reached before the seventh week in more than half the cases, only a few remaining patients with EP will benefit from the conventional, transabdominal sonographic examination.

Transvaginal sonography (TVS) is certain to overcome some of these limitations because of the high-resolution transducer and the conjecture that proximity to structures is involved in the process of diagnosing ectopic gestation.

INVASIVE DIAGNOSIS OF ECTOPIC PREGNANCY

The "invasive" diagnostic procedures for diagnosing an ectopic pregnancy are the *D&C, culdocentesis,* and *laparoscopy.*

In a "stable" patient with vaginal bleeding, an undefined intrauterine finding on transabdominal sonography, and a serum HCG level lower than 6,500 mIU/mL and where the pregnancy is unwanted, a D&C may help confirm the diagnosis.[17] For its historical merit, culdocentesis must be mentioned here. This invasive technique is losing popularity because of its high false-positive rate in cases of bleeding ovarian cysts as well as its high false-negative rate in cases of unruptured "early" ectopic pregnancy; it is being replaced by noninvasive sonography coupled with β-HCG determination.

Laparoscopy, the third and last of the invasive techniques used to diagnose ectopic gestation, is well established; its use in diagnosing tubal pregnancies will continue until sonographic diagnosis becomes more reliable. The advantage of laparoscopy is its versatility. In cases of unruptured tubal gestation, the diagnostic procedure can continue as a therapeutic–surgical one. The need for hospitalization and anesthesia should not deter the managing team. Despite its high accuracy, laparoscopy may miss the diagnosis of a pregnancy if the Fallopian tube is only slightly distended by a 0.5-cm gestational sac, or if technical difficulties are encountered in viewing the tubes, even though the false-positive and false-negative rates are low, both being about 3%.

The use of laparoscopy becomes extremely important in surgical management if an unruptured tubal gestation is diagnosed and the patient desires future pregnancies.[20] In the last few years, conservative laparoscopic procedures have been performed to extract the products of conception while preserving the tube.

USE OF THE TRANSVAGINAL PROBE IN THE WORKUP OF ECTOPIC PREGNANCY

If possible, the sonographic workup should always start with a transvaginal scan. If the urinary bladder of the patient is full, one may proceed first to abdominal scanning. As mentioned before, a slightly reversed Trendelenburg position should be maintained throughout the examination.

A systematic approach is advised. Scan the uterus first, then the Fallopian tube and the cul-de-sac, and, finally, look for rare but possible alternate sites of an ectopic gestation.

The procedures to be performed are discussed below in detail:

Uterus

Intrauterine Pregnancies. Intrauterine pregnancies can be documented with absolute reliability as early as 5 weeks from the LMP, regardless of patient obesity or position of the uterus. Very early imaging of embryonic and extraembryonic structures enhances the reliability of diagnosing a normal or abnormal intrauterine gestation. (For a detailed description the reader is referred to Chapters 6 and 7.) Once intrauterine pregnancy has been diagnosed, one may, with high confidence, discard the suspicion of ectopic pregnancy.

Endometrial Response to Extrauterine Pregnancy. The endometrium responds to adequate hormonal stimulation of the growing extrauterine gestation. Transvaginal sonography may demonstrate a highly echogenic, thickened endometrium. Eventually the ectopic and immature trophoblast ceases to secrete, leading to decidual degeneration and bleeding (Fig. 8.1). This bleeding may have been what various authors[21-23] described as the "pseudogestational sac" (PGS) of ectopic pregnancy. This PGS is primarily located symmetrically in the center of the uterus, outlining its cavity. If TVS detects an ectopic gestation early enough (at a time when no decidual degeneration has yet occurred), no intracavital bleeding occurs. Hence no pseudogestational sac should be seen. Later,

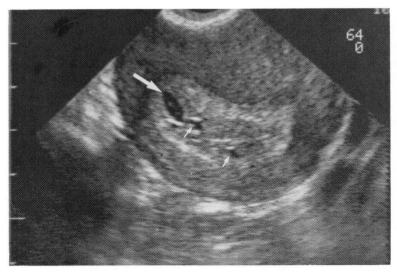

FIGURE 8.1 Transverse section of the uterus in a case of ectopic gestation. Note the thick endometrium with a clearly defined sonolucent area (large arrow) that is devoid of the decidual double ring of a normal gestation. The cavity line (small arrows) is marked by small sonolucent structures all of which may represent bleeding. The patient had vaginal spotting.

as mentioned earlier, hormonal support of the endometrium decreases and occult intracavital bleeding is imminent. Therefore, it is our feeling that this concealed bleeding was defined in classic transabdominal examinations as the pseudogestational sac. Appearance of this PGS may precede overt vaginal bleeding by several hours or days.

A *normal* or *true gestational sac* must show two distinct features easily demonstrated by TVS: first, a *double-contoured gestational sac* previously described by transabdominal sonography[23,24]; second, peculiar lacunar structures with a distinct flow appearing at one pole of the gestational sac (Fig 8.2**a**). These structures have not yet been described by others in the sonographic literature.[25] The lacunar formations can be demonstrated only by TVS and may be forerunners of the placental site. We believe that maternal blood flow to the site of implantation produces this picture. This flow was seen to persist around the gestational sac for several days after cessation of a previously detected fetal heartbeat in the case of abnormal gestations. If a pseudogestational sac was observed, no such flow could be visualized by transvaginal sonography. We had the impression that in a small number of tubal gestations these lacunar "lakes" showing blood flow could be seen (Fig 8.2**b**).

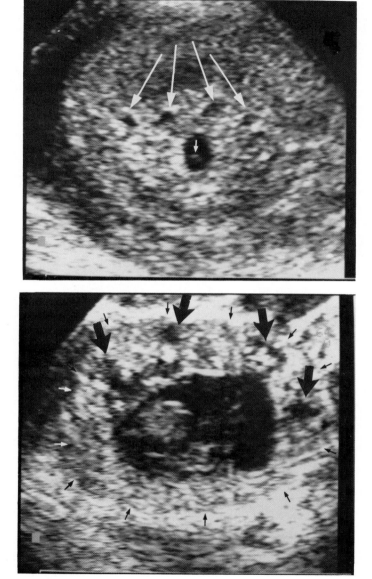

A

B

FIGURE 8.2 (**a**) A 5-week 2-day *intrauterine* gestation; the small arrow points to the yolk sac. The four long arrows point to lacunal structures. During real-time scan, flow is seen in these places. (**b**) Cross section of the Fallopian tube at the level of the ampulla outlined by small arrows. Tubal wall is "invaded" by a trophoblast. Lacunar structures (large arrows) showing flow under real time can be observed. The gestational sac contains a live embryo (7 weeks gestation from the LMP).

Fallopian Tube

The Progressing Tubal Pregnancy. In the case of a live tubal pregnancy, the embryo will continue to grow until the tubal epithelium is able to "sustain" the already implanted sac. The similarity between the lacunar (maternal?) blood flow of a very early tubal gestation and the previously described lacunar blood flow of an intrauterine gestation (Fig 8.2**b**) is worth mentioning. In this early stage, development of the embryo and extraembryonic structures is similar to that in intrauterine gestation. The ectopic gestational sac with a visible heartbeat, adjacent to the fetal pole, is revealed by transvaginal scanning (Figs 8.3 and 8.4). The advantage of the high-frequency transvaginal probe lies in its ability to visualize a live tubal pregnancy before its rupture or before tubal abortion occurs. Em-

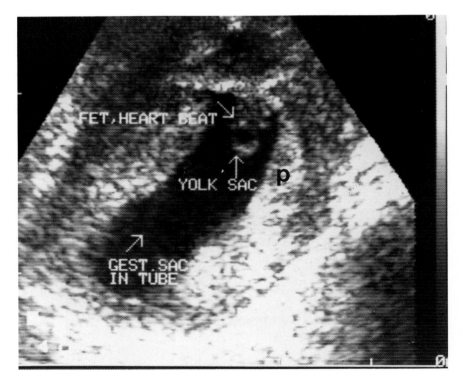

FIGURE 8.3 Longitudinal section of the right tube containing gestational sac, fetal pole, yolk sac, and placenta (p). Heartbeats were seen on the real-time scan. Unruptured tubal pregnancy was confirmed by laparoscopy (6 weeks 4 days from the LMP).

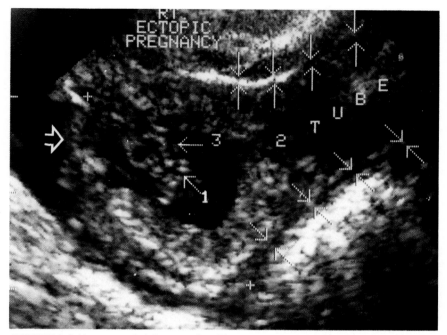

FIGURE 8.4 Unruptured right ampullar (2) pregnancy, 6 weeks 3 days from the LMP. Fetal pole (1) and yolk sac (3) are evident. Arrows point to tubal contours. The open arrow points to the distal end of the tube (fimbrioplasty was performed 20 months prior to this ectopic pregnancy).

bryonic structures, such as the fetal pole with heartbeats, or extraembryonic structures, such as the yolk sac and the tiny placenta, may be recognized by the attentive sonographer (Figs 8.2–8.5). Once the diagnosis of tubal gestation has been made, exact location of the cyesis along the tube may be attempted (Fig 8.3).

During an analysis of cases of tubal pregnancy in which the diagnosis had been made by transvaginal sonography, it was noted that in each and every case of *unruptured* tubal pregnancy (*with or without* the detection of fetal heartbeats) the tubal wall containing the sac was thickened, measuring 4–6 mm (Figs 8.2b, 8.3–8.7). As against the term "adnexal ring" used in TAS, we propose the more precise description *tubal ring*.

Tubal Abortion. The ectopic and immature trophoblast in the tube may not secrete adequate quantities of HCG to sustain a normal corpus luteum. Corpus luteum insufficiency occurs and the embryo dies.

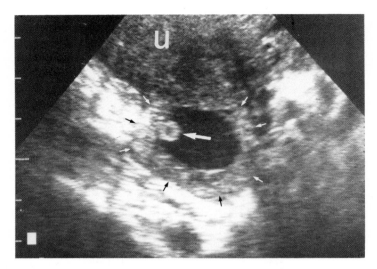

FIGURE 8.5 Cross section of an intact left tube (note its thick wall marked by small arrows) containing the gestational sac was visualized in the cul-de-sac below the uterus (u). This section shows the yolk sac (large arrow). The fetal pole with heartbeats was seen on a subsequent section.

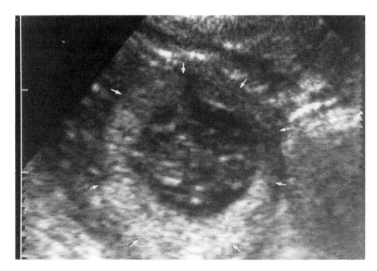

FIGURE 8.6 Cross section of the right salpinx is outlined by arrows. An irregularly echogenic substance was noted to fill its lumen. At surgery, a blood clot was extracted, along with the products of conception, from the unruptured ampullar section of the tube.

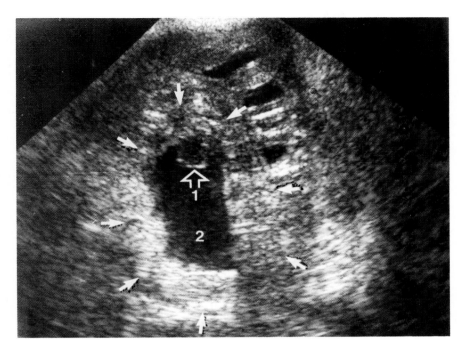

FIGURE 8.7 Arrows outline the cross section of a tube with gestational sac (2). The open arrow (1) points to the shrunken, amorphous fetal pole. No heartbeats were observed in this 6½-week ectopic gestation.

Development of the "tubal embryo" is dependent not only on the levels of secreted hormones but also on the trophoblast's ability to "invade" the underlying tissue to ensure blood support. Since this trophoblast will not be able to find an adequate decidual–placental bed, it will have to invade the muscular wall of the tube. This muscular wall is then weakened and eroded by the ingrowing chorionic tissue in search of supporting blood vessels. The stretching and erosion of the tubal wall result in bleeding into the sac as well as between the tubal wall and the gestational sac.

Once the gestational sac has separated from the tubal wall, four events may occur[26]:

1. Rupture of the sac into the lumen of the tube (Fig 8.6).

2. Absorption of the gestation (Fig 8.7).

3. Abortion into the pelvis (extrusion of the ectopic gestation through the

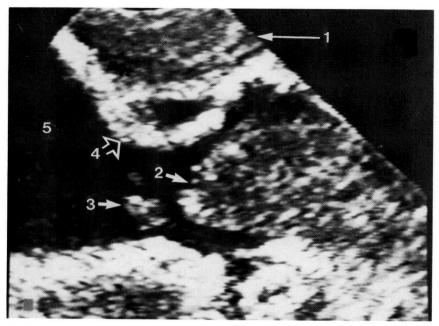

FIGURE 8.8 In the cul-de-sac, behind the uterus (1), a thickened left tube (2) containing blood clots floats in free fluid (5). Adhesions are seen emerging from the posterior aspect of the uterus (4). Thin fimbriae (3) are near the distal end of the tube. Laparoscopy confirmed the sonographic finding of tubal abortion.

fimbrial end into the peritoneal cavity). If this occurs, the thickened tubal wall may be seen in the blood collecting into the pelvis (Fig 8.8).

4. A slow blood leak or rupture of the tube leading to pelvic intraperitoneal fluid collection.

Cul-de-sac

Careful examination of the space posterior to the uterus may provide us with two important pieces of information:

(a) The *presence* of *free fluid* in an amount larger than normally detected, with or without blood clots (Fig 8.9). The blood clots are depicted as a bizarre-shaped mass of irregularly echogenic substance. They may float freely; thin chords of fibrin are attached to their surface. If the

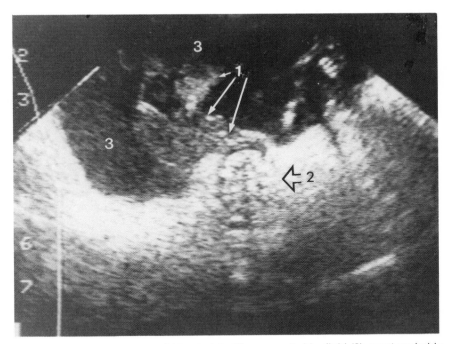

FIGURE 8.9 Irregularly shaped blood clots (1) surrounded by fluid (3), most probably blood, in the Douglas space anterior to the cross section of the rectum (2).

probe is gently moved in and out or the patient is asked to tilt her pelvis to the right and the left several times, the blood clots may be observed to move. When free fluid is detected one may search the tubes for more detailed information concerning the presence or absence of the tubal contents. As described in Chapter 2, this fluid creates optimal contrast for visualization of the tube, improving diagnostic accuracy. The importance of placing the patient in a reversed Trendelenburg position cannot be overstressed. If the patient can stand up, she should do so and wait about 1 minute before assuming the proper position for the transvaginal scan. The examiner should patiently wait longer in anticipation of a possible slow appearance of fluid before making the diagnosis that "no free fluid was detected in the pelvis."

(b) *The absence of free fluid* excludes the possibility of active bleeding into the pelvis. In this case, the sonographer's attention must be directed to the uterus and the tubes as well as to other clinical and laboratory data to provide evidence for or rule out EP.

Other Possible Sites for EP

Bear in mind that a small fraction of ectopic pregnancies are located in the ovaries, uterine cervix, pelvis, or abdomen. It is believed that even with high-frequency transvaginal sonography, their detection will continue to present serious problems to the sonographer.

HOW CAN TRANSVAGINAL SONOGRAPHY HELP IN THE DIAGNOSIS AND MANAGEMENT OF ECTOPIC PREGNANCY?

Obviously, the diagnostic power of the transvaginal probe in general, and the 6.5-MHz probe in particular, lies in the superior imaging resulting from the high resolution. The diagnosis or exclusion of an ectopic gestation depends heavily on a combination of two or more of the following features:

Documentation of the Intrauterine Pregnancy and Extraembryonic Structures at a Very Early Stage

1. Appearance of the gestational sac at less than 5 weeks from the LMP.
2. Early diagnosis of the typical double ring of a normal gestation with lacunar flow adjacent to the gestation (described in Chapter 6).
3. Appearance and outlining of the yolk sac 5 weeks from the LMP.
4. Detection of fetal heartbeats as early as 6 weeks from the LMP.

Exclusion of Intrauterine Pregnancy by Documentation of the Lack of a Gestational Sac in the Uterus

In other words, TVS makes it possible to distinguish between a true gestational sac and an endometrial response to an ectopic gestation (eg, pseudogestational sac). Although it occurs rarely, a concomitant intrauterine and extrauterine pregnancy should always be kept in mind and ruled out.

Documentation of Tubal Pregnancy

Imaging the typical "tubal ring" in cases of unruptured tubal EP is of the utmost importance. Embryonic structures (fetal pole, fetal heartbeats) and extraembryonic structures (yolk sac, cord, membranes, trophoblastic layers) are recognized with a great deal of accuracy in cases of progressing unruptured tubal gestation.

Fluid in Cul-de-sac

Precise and reliable evaluation of the cul-de-sac for presence or absence
of fluid, with or without blood clots, is an important component of the
diagnostic algorithm in cases of "leaking," unruptured, and/or ruptured
tubal gestations.

Tubal Pathology Other Than Tubal Pregnancy

A dependable diagnosis of tubal conditions other than tubal pregnancy
may readily be made, excluding them from the list of different diagnoses.
These and other pathological findings are bound to add confusion to the
diagnosis of EP. The list is long; some of the possibilities are corpus
luteum hemorrhage or cyst, tubo-ovarian abscess, hydrosalpinx,
pyosalpinx, and torsion of the ovarian cyst. These are described in different chapters of this book.

Despite the fact that one would very much like to diagnose and treat
EP in its early stages, the final diagnosis is often made in emergency
situations after intraperitoneal bleeding occurs. To avoid these emergency situations, invasive diagnostic techniques such as culdocentesis,
endometrial curettage, laparoscopy, and laparotomy are liberally applied.
On the basis of our experience in this field, we feel that in addition to a
rapidly available serum β-HCG test for serial titrations, the use of transvaginal sonography will in the near future reduce the use of the above-
mentioned, sometimes superfluous, invasive diagnostic procedures. This
prediction, of course, is based on early and clear images of pelvic anatomy and pathology.

The potential diagnostic accuracy of TVS in detection of an ectopic
gestation in its incipient stages enables early and elective, as well as
relatively minor, surgical intervention, eg, translaparoscopic removal of
the small ovisac.[20,27] The alternative is rushing the patient later to a major
and more extensive emergency surgery. In the case of a *missed tubal
pregnancy,* the conservative follow-up of a gradually resorbing gestation
can be made by the transvaginal sonographic approach.

The authors have considered the possibility of applying the combined
techniques of transvaginal follicle aspiration and ultrasound-guided puncture for early first-trimester reduction in the number of fetuses in cases of
multiple pregnancies[28,29] and for the treatment of unruptured tubal gestation. Feichtinger and Kemeter[30] have pioneered this semi-invasive puncture procedure, treating an unruptured tubal gestation by injecting 10 mg
of methotrexate in 1 mL of solution after aspirating the fluid contents of
the gestational sac. Levels of β-HCG dropped to 0, and tubal patency was

demonstrated by a subsequent hysterosalpingogram (W. Feichtinger and P. Kemeter, personal communication).

Finally, the practical and clinical yield of early detection of ectopic pregnancy by transvaginal sonography has two important elements:

1. Further reduction of maternal mortality and morbidity.
2. Conservation of future fertility for patients desiring further childbearing.

Although more meaningful studies with statistical support are still in progress, we feel that the high-frequency transvaginal transducer will soon become the main tool in the early diagnosis of ectopic gestation.

REFERENCES

1. Sivin I, Cooper T: IUD use and ectopic pregnancy rates in the United States. Contraception 1979;19:151–173.
2. Rubin GL, Peterson HB, Dorfman SF, et al: Ectopic pregnancy in the United States, 1970 through 1978. JAMA 1983;249:1725–1729.
3. Westrom L, Bengtsson L, Mardh PA: Incidence, trends and risks of ectopic pregnancy in a population of women. Br Med J 1981;282:15–18.
4. Tancer ML, Delke I, Veridiano NP: A fifteen year experience with ectopic pregnancy. Surg Gynecol Obstet 1981;152:179–183.
5. Hazelkamp JT: Ectopic pregnancy: Diagnostic dilemma and delay. Int J Gynaecol Obstet 1980;17:598–601.
6. Curran JW: Economic consequences of pelvic inflammatory disease in the United States. Am J Obstet Gynecol 1980;138:848–851.
7. Schwartz RD, DiPietro DL: BHCG as a diagnostic aid for suspected ectopic pregnancy. Obstet Gynecol 1980;56:197–201.
8. Derman R, Edelman DA, Berger GS: Current status of immunologic pregnancy tests. Int J Gynaecol Obstet 1979;17:190–198.
9. Jacobson E, Rothe D: False positive hemagglutination tests for pregnancy with tuboovarian abscess. Int J Gynaecol Obstet 1980;17:307–312.
10. Rasor FL, Braunstein GD: A rapid modification of the BHCG radioimmunoassay. Use as an aid in the diagnosis of ectopic pregnancy. Obstet Gynecol 1977;50:553–557.
11. Vaitukaitis FL, Braunstein GD, Ross GT: Radioimmunoassay which specifically measures human chorionic gonadotrophin in the presence of luteinizing hormone. Am J Obstet Gynecol 1972;113:751–758.
12. Seppala M, Tontiti K, Ranta T, et al: Use of a rapid hCG beta-subunit radioimmunoassay in acute gynaecological emergencies. Lancet 1980;1:165–167.
13. Ackerman R, Deutsch S, Krumholtz B: Levels of human chorionic gonadotropin in unruptured and ruptured ectopic pregnancy. Obstet Gynecol 1982;60:13–16.
14. Kadar N, Taylor KJW, Rosenfield AT: Combined use of serum HCG and sonography in the diagnosis of ectopic pregnancy. Am J Roentgenol 1983;141:609–615.
15. Lawson, TL: Ectopic pregnancy, criteria and accuracy of ultrasonic diagnosis. Am J Roentgenol 1978;131:153–158.

16. Brown TW, Filly RA, Laing FC, et al: Analysis of ultrasonographic criteria in the evaluation for ectopic pregnancy. Am J Roentgenol 1978;131:967–971.
17. Kadar N, DeVore G, Romero R: Discriminatory HCG zone. Its use in sonographic evaluation for ectopic pregnancy. Obstet Gynecol 1981;58:156–161.
18. Nyberg DA, Filly RA, Mahoney BS, et al: Correlation of HCG levels and sonographic identification. Am J Roentgenol 1985;144:951–954.
19. Levi S, Leblicq P: The diagnostic value of ultrasonography in 342 suspected cases of ectopic pregnancy. Acta Obstet Gynecol Scand 1980;59:29–36.
20. Stangel J: Newer methods of treatment of ectopic pregnancy, in De Cherney AH (ed): Ectopic Pregnancy. Rockville, Md, Aspen Publishers Inc, 1986, pp 89–102.
21. Weiner C: The pseudogestational sac in ectopic pregnancy. Am J Obstet Gynecol 1981;139:959–961.
22. Abramovici H, Auslender R, Lewin A, et al: Gestational–pseudogestational sac: A new ultrasonic criterion for differential diagnosis. Am J Obstet Gynecol 1983;145:377–379.
23. Nyberg DA, Laing FC, Filly RA, et al: Ultrasonic differentiation of the gestational sac of early pregnancy from the pseudogestational sac of ectopic pregnancy. Radiology 1978;146:755–759.
24. Bradley WC, Fiske CE, Filly RA: The double sac sign of early intrauterine pregnancy: Use in exclusion of ectopic pregnancy. Radiology 1982;143:223–226.
25. Timor-Tritsch IE, Rottem S: Transvaginal sonographic study of the Fallopian tube. Gynecol Obstet, in press.
26. Parsons L, Sommers SC: Ectopic Pregnancy in Gynecology. Philadelphia, WB Saunders Co, 1978, pp 500–526.
27. De Cherney AH, Romero R, Naftolin F: Surgical management of unruptured ectopic pregnancy. Fertil Steril 1981;35:21–24.
28. Bessis R, Milanese C, Frydman R: Preventive partial termination in multiple pregnancy. Presented at the Second International Symposium: The Fetus as a Patient—Diagnosis and Therapy. Israel, May 26, 1985.
29. Vrijens R, Beckhuizen W, Rombant R: Selective interruption of multiple pregnancy by ultrasonographic guidance, in Proceedings of the World Congress of the World Federation of Ultrasound in Medicine and Biology. Sydney, Australia, 1985, p 271.
30. Feichtinger W, Kemeter P: Conservative treatment of ectopic pregnancy by transvaginal aspiration under sonographic control and methotrexate injection. Lancet, 1987;1:381.

CHAPTER 9

The Use of Transvaginal Sonography in Infertility

Arieh Drugan, MD, Zeev Blumenfeld, MD,
Yochanan Erlik, MD, Ilan E. Timor-Tritsch, MD,
and Joseph M. Brandes, MD

Infertility is a major problem affecting 15–20% of married couples. About 40–50% of affected couples suffer from problems of oligo-anovulation; about 15% of infertile women suffer from mechanical infertility, and a substantial proportion of them require in vitro fertilization (IVF). Therefore, it seems that about 5–10% of the female population require induction of ovulation.

For years, ovulation was monitored entirely by clinical parameters. Later, with the advent of radioimmunoassay, hormonal parameters were the predominant tool used for evaluation of ovulation induction.

The use of ultrasound in the diagnosis and treatment of female infertility was introduced in the report of Kratochwil et al[1] on visualization of pelvic organs. Later, Hackeloer et al[2] correlated follicular size determined by ultrasound (U/S) with 17 β-estradiol (E_2) measurements. Ultrasound-guided collection of human oocytes for IVF was introduced in 1981 by Lenz et al[3]; as they and others further improved the technique, the results of ultrasound-guided oocyte retrieval came to equal those of the more "traditional" method, laparoscopy.[4] Gleicher et al[5] in 1983 and later Dellenbach et al[6] in 1984 introduced the transvaginal approach to oocyte retrieval for IVF.

In this chapter we report our experience with transvaginal sonographic monitoring, with a 6.5-MHz transducer probe, of ovulation induction in relation to the ovarian and endometrial cycles and we describe the method used by us for TVS-guided transvaginal oocyte retrieval.

The transvaginal route was at first preferred in obese patients in whom tissue attenuation prevents the efficient use of the abdominal transducer. More recently, because of the closeness of the transducer probe to the pelvic organs and the high resolution of the pictures obtained, this technique has been used in many centers. TVS is preferred because it provides (a) maximal clarity of the ovaries, the uterus, and the pelvic blood vessels as well as the follicular borders, and (b) patient convenience and compliance, since a full bladder is not necessary for the examination.

MONITORING OF OVULATION INDUCTION

Ovarian Cycle

Follicles can be pictured starting at a diameter of 3–5 mm, but they reach clinical importance starting at a diameter of 10 mm. This occurs approximately at day 6 or, in other words, 6 days before evidence of ovulation. Later on in the natural ovarian cycle, usually only one follicle dominates. Hackeloer et al[2,7,8] found that the rate of growth of the dominant follicle was linear from day 5 to ovulation, with an average daily growth rate of 2 mm. The mean diameters of the follicle before ovulation ranged between 18 and 24 mm (average 20.2 mm). They also found that the amount of estrogen produced by a single follicle increases as the follicle matures, and there is a linear correlation between follicular diameter and E_2 level in serum.[2] This observation correlated well with those of Baird and Fraser,[9] who demonstrated that 95% of the circulating E_2 emanates from the growing dominant follicle. De Cherney and Laufer[10] surveyed the literature and found that in the natural cycle, ovulation occurs within a narrow range of follicular diameters (20–25 mm). Compared with E_2 level, follicular size (as estimated by U/S) was more accurate in predicting ovulation, although better timing of ovulation was achieved by using both parameters. In induced cycles, using ovulation induction agents like clomiphene citrate or human menopausal gonadotropins, generally more than one dominant follicle developed. In this case, although serum E_2 level and sonographically measured follicular growth seemed to increase linearly, the correlation between these two parameters was significantly lower than in the natural cycle. It seems that total follicular volume shows the highest correlation with serum E_2 in induced cycles, as the rate of growth of the individual follicle and the leading follicle can change during the cycle.[11] In the induced cycle, the value of ultrasonography is in making the decision to withhold administration of HCG when E_2 levels are apparently ovulatory, deriving from the development of multiple but small follicles.[10] As

Siebel et al showed, premature administration of HCG at a follicular diameter smaller than 14 mm resulted in atresia of the follicles and a short luteal phase.[12]

Technique of Follicular Measurement

In studies of follicular development, sector scanners are preferred to linear scanners. Follicular development is studied using real-time gray-scale sector scanners. The Elscint ESI 1000 equipped with a 6.5-MHz transvaginal transducer was employed. Technical data for the transducer were described in Chapter 1.

The procedure is performed with the patient in the lithotomy position after she has emptied her bladder. A more detailed step-by-step description of the technique is given in Chapter 2. The midline plane with the uterus must be visualized first. Introducing the transducer deep into the vagina and pointing it to one of the sides, one measures and examines the ovary and its follicles. Anatomical landmarks may be employed to locate the ovaries. In addition to the uterus representing the "midline" of the pelvis, one may use a clearly visible lateral structure: iliac vein and artery. Flow and pulsation can be recognized in these two vessels.

Figures 9.1a–9.1d show and compare follicles observed transabdominally and transvaginally.

Follicular volume is measured using the formula

$$volume = 11 \times A \times B \times C$$

(the follicle being an ovoid, A, B, and C are the largest diameters measured on three planes). When only two dimensions or two planes are available, the formula that should be used is

$$volume = 11 \times A \times B \times B$$

(where A is the largest and B is the smallest diameter measured).

A few anatomical structures may look similar to the ovarian follicle. These include (1) the cross section of the internal iliac artery and vein, (2) the cross section of blood vessels around the uterus and the ovary, (3) the bowel, (4) the hydrosalpinx, and (5) ovarian cysts.

Vessels can usually be distinguished by their pulsatility and by changing the transducer scanning plane by 90°. The round structure previously observed changes to an elongated one (two parallel lines) with or without pulsation. Parts of the bowel, if looked at for several seconds, show peristalsis, and the intraluminal contents are generally somewhat echogenic. Hydrosalpinges and ovarian cysts are more difficult to distinguish

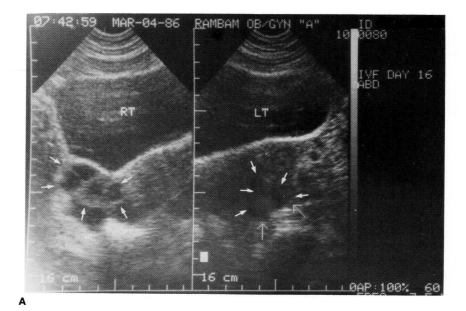

A

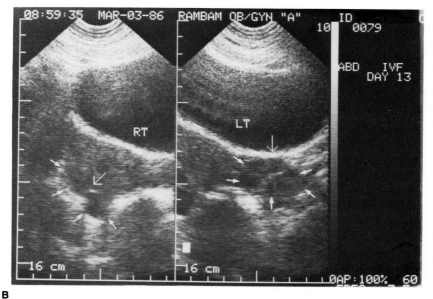

B

FIGURE 9.1 Comparison of views of ovarian follicles by the transabdominal/transvesical route (**a,b**) and the transvaginal route (**c,d**). Both patients' ovaries were hormonally stimulated and scanned on the day of ovulation induction.

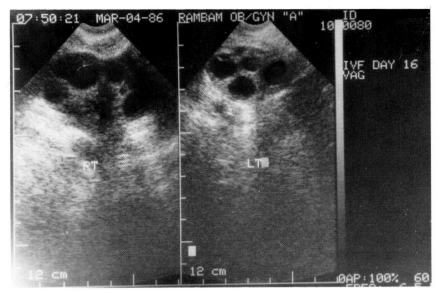

C

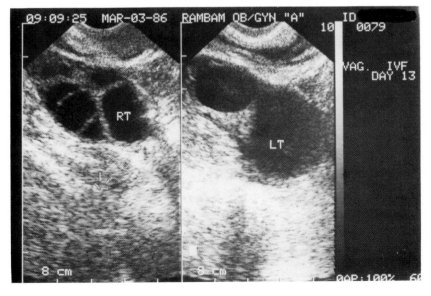

D

structurally from larger follicles. In such cases, serial daily scanning helps, as these structures do not grow much under the influence of hormonal treatment.

Ovulatory and postovulatory events may also be seen. Because of its mucoid consistency, the cumulus mass can be observed in about 60–65% of preovulatory follicles, 12–24 hours before ovulation[2] (Fig 9.2). De Crespigny et al[13] observed ovulatory events and showed that for a period of up to 7 hours prior to ovulation there was no change in the size or appearance of the follicle. This period was followed by release of antral fluid and collapse of the follicle, a sudden event that can be very quick or take up to 35 minutes. A corpus hemorrhagicum (filling of the follicle area with echogenic material) was seen to develop during the next hour or so. The expelled fluid collects in the cul-de-sac (Fig 3.7); this ultrasonographic finding, together with echogenic areas and blurring of the follicular borders, is accepted as evidence of ovulation. However, the observer must remember that some fluid may be seen in the cul-de-sac even before ovulation. This fluid seems to be caused by transudation from the dominant follicle. Figures 9.3**a** and 9.3**b** show the development of the corpus luteum as seen by TVS.

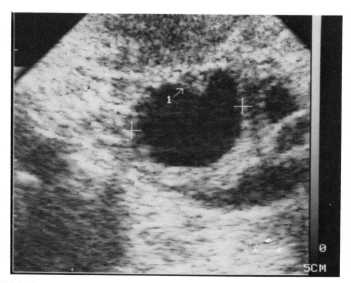

FIGURE 9.2 Preovulatory follicle; arrow points to cumulus mass.

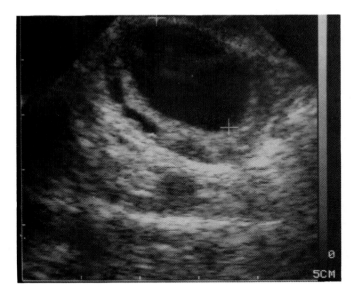

A

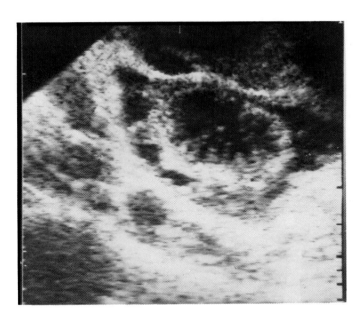

B

FIGURE 9.3 Corpus luteum formation. (**a**) Dominant follicle on day 15 in an unstimula-
ted cycle. (**b**) Same ovary 3 days later. Note wheel–spike appearance of intrafollicular
hemorrhage: corpus luteum.

Endometrial Cycle

The endometrium represents an end organ for circulating estrogens and, therefore, provides a useful assay of changing hormonal levels. With the use of advanced ultrasound technology and expertise, serial changes in the endometrium can be detected through the stimulated menstrual cycle. Two aspects of the endometrium appear to change progressively throughout the preovulatory phase: reflectivity and thickness. Smith et al[14] described reflectivity as a means of endometrial grading based on comparison of the gray-scale appearance of endometrial texture with that of myometrial texture. Four patterns of endometrial response can be distinguished as described by transabdominal sonography:

Grade D is characterized by an almost anechogenic endometrium in the presence of a prominent midline echo. This endometrial pattern is commonly seen in the early to midfollicular phase and is considered the least favorable.

Grade C is characterized by a solid area of reduced reflectivity and therefore appears darker than the surrounding myometrium. This is a mild but positive response to increasing levels of circulating E_2.

Grade B endometrium is comparable in reflectivity to the surrounding myometrium and its gray-scale appearance is indistinguishable. The initial appearance of an endometrial halo is notable. This pattern represents a good endometrial response.

Grade A endometrium appears brighter than the myometrium.

The thickness of the endometrium is measured on both sides of the midline, through the central longitudinal axis of the uterine body. Increasing thickness of the endometrium is associated with higher levels of E_2, with more mature oocytes, and with higher rates of fertilization and pregnancy. An endometrial thickness less than 5 mm is usually associated with an immature phase of the follicular cycle. Closer to the time of ovulation or at ovulation, a grade A endometrium with an approximate thickness of 10 mm is expected.

Because of its higher resolution the transvaginal transducer makes possible detection and measurement of the above-mentioned endometrial cycles with greater precision. Representative pictures are shown in Figure 9.4.

FIGURE 9.4 Example of a transvaginal ultrasonographic view of endometrial response. (a) Transverse section of uterus with endometrial response grade C. (b) Longitudinal section of the same uterus. (*continued*)

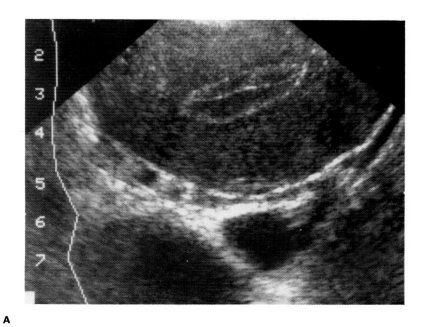

A

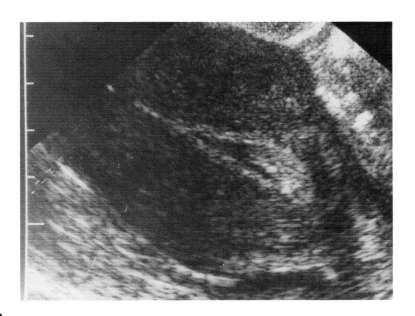

B

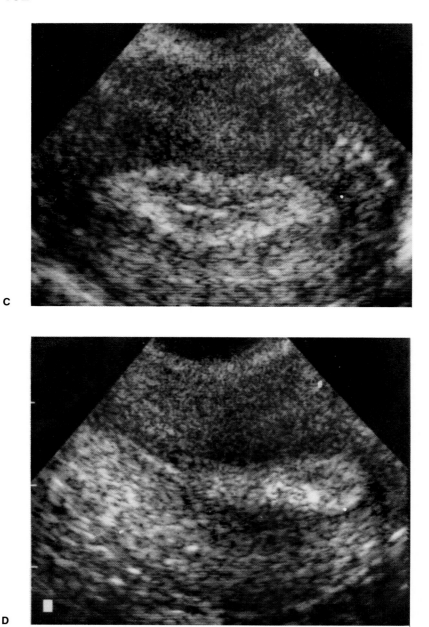

FIGURE 9.4 (*continued*) (**c**) Transverse section of a uterus with endometrial response grade A. (**d**) Longitudinal section of the same endometrium.

TRANSVAGINAL ULTRASONOGRAPHY-GUIDED OOCYTE RETRIEVAL FOR IN VITRO FERTILIZATION AND EMBRYO TRANSFER

Ultrasound-guided follicle puncture for IVF/ET was introduced by Lenz et al in 1981.[3] As the procedure may be performed in an ambulatory setup, the cost of the cycle and the risks of general anesthesia are minimized. This is also the reason for its increasing popularity. With expertise, as well as with continuous improvements in the equipment, the results of this method have become comparable to those of laparoscopic ovum retrieval.

The transvesical approach is sometimes difficult to perform because the ovaries are located deep in the cul-de-sac or the patient has a thick, obese abdominal wall.[15,16]

The transvaginal approach to oocyte retrieval was introduced by Dellenbach et al[6] (1984), who used transvesical ultrasonographic guidance. In 1986, Kemeter and Feichtinger[17] reported their experience with transvaginal oocyte retrieval using a transvaginal sector scan probe combined with an automated puncture device. Their latest statistics[18] show a 98.3% TVS oocyte retrieval rate in 61 patients, with an average of 4.5 oocytes aspirated per patient (slightly higher than the 3.6 ova per patient obtained with the transabdominal ultrasound-guided procedures performed by the same group on 371 patients). More comparative statistics are given in Table 9.1, which is compiled from their data. It seems that the IVF/ET statistics on patients in whom transvaginal sonographic guidance was used were comparable to, or slightly better than, those on patients approached abdominally.

Another "transvaginal technique" is currently in use: transvaginal needle puncture of the follicle guided with a transabdominal transducer probe.[19] This technique can be dangerous, yielding a low rate of oocyte retrieval (2.2 per procedure); also, the only two cases of laceration of the iliac veins reported occurred when this technique was used.[19] The probable reasons for this complication are (1) the lack of alignment of the scanning plane and "freehand"-operated vaginally inserted needle (thus, the tip of the needle is not seen on the screen and may inadvertently sever the large pelvic vessel), and (2) the requirement of a full bladder with the transabdominally operated transducer. A full bladder creates pressure on the ovaries, pressing them closer against the pelvic floor, closer to the iliac vein and the rectum.

Considering that the needle guides attached to the probe are available, and that the advancing needle can be controlled throughout the entire procedure with the parallel-placed vaginal transducer, the above-

TABLE 9.1 Comparison of Transabdominal versus Transvaginal
Ultrasound-Guided Aspiration of Oocytes

	Follicle Aspiration by Transabdominal Ultrasound Guidance	Follicle Aspiration by Transvaginal Ultrasound Guidance
Attempted oocyte recoveries	371	61
Successful oocyte recoveries	351 (94.6%)	60 (98.3%)
Follicles (2 mL)	1,568	323
Oocytes	1,345 (85.8%)	278 (86%)
Average oocytes per oocyte recovery	3.6	4.5
Fertilized oocytes	796 (59.2%)	176 (63.3%)
Embryo replacements	252 (68%)	49 (80.3%)
Clinical pregnancies	46 (12.4% PCT,[a] 18.2% ER)	13 (21.3% PCT, 26.5% ER)
Abortions	8	4
Ectopic pregnancies	4	0
Normal pregnancies and deliveries	34 (9.2% PCT, 13.5% ER)	9 (14.7% PCT, 18.3% ER)

Adapted from Feichtinger and Kemeter.[18]
[a] PCT = puncture, ER = embryo replacement.

mentioned combination abdominal–vaginal approach should be considered obsolete and harmful.

TRANSVAGINAL ASPIRATION PROCEDURE

The transvaginal oocyte retrieval procedure has been used at the Rambam Medical Center since 1985.

The vaginal transducer probe is fitted with a needle guide (Fig 9.5). The aspiration needle is advanced along the software-generated penetration line observed on the screen. The patient is prepared for the procedure as follows: Povidone-iodine (Polydine, Fisher) vaginal suppositories are employed the day before and the day of follicular aspiration to obtain a sterile vaginal mucosa. The patient is placed in the lithotomy position after she voluntarily empties her bladder. First, transvaginal ultrasound scanning is performed to locate the follicles (Fig 9.6) and cul-de-sac to rule out ovulation. Then, the vagina is thoroughly cleaned again with povidone-iodine solution and rinsed with sterile normal saline. The patient is draped with sterile covers, sterile polyethylene sheets are placed

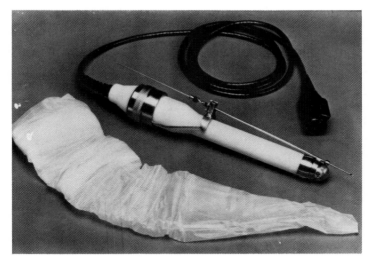

FIGURE 9.5 Transvaginal 6.5-MHz transducer fitted with guide, needle, and sterile probe covers.

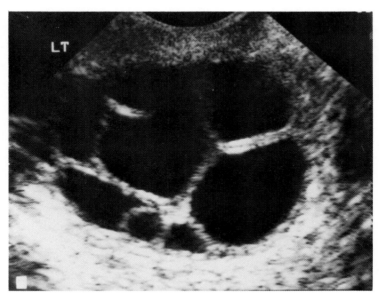

FIGURE 9.6 Cross section of left ovary after hormonal induction of ovulation before oocyte retrieval. Note how the high resolution of the 6.5-MHz probe enables visualization of each and every follicle with its follicular wall.

on the keyboard of the scanner, and the transducer is slipped into a sterile bag. Pethidine (Demerol) HCl, 50–150 mg, and diazepam (Valium, Roche), 10–15 mg, are administered intravenously to induce relaxation or a short sleep.

The transducer is then introduced deep into the vagina, and the largest diameter of the target follicle is aligned with the biopsy line. The follicle is entered with a 25-cm-long, 1.4-mm-internal-diameter stainless steel needle (Izmel Ltd., Israel) and the follicular fluid is aspirated (Fig 9.7), under a suction pressure of 100 mm Hg, into a sterile culture flask (Falcon No. 2037) containing 1 mL of Dulbeco's phosphate-buffered saline. The follicle is flushed again with culture medium and is seen to enlarge as flushing fluid is injected. Turbulence is evident from the echogenic properties of the micro-air bubbles containing flushing fluid (Fig 9.8). It is our impression that the collapse of the follicle is much faster if the vaginal aspiration method is used as opposed to the abdominal aspira-

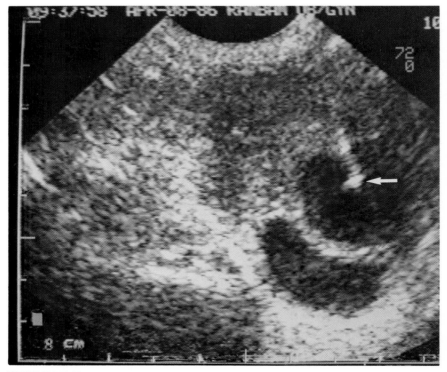

FIGURE 9.7 Follicular aspiration; the needle tip is seen inside the follicle (arrow).

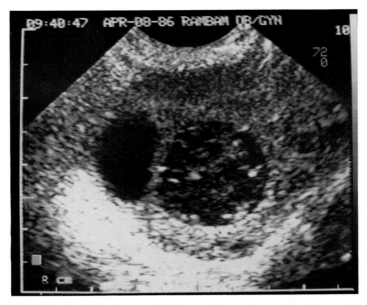

FIGURE 9.8 Follicular flush; turbulent fluid containing micro-air bubbles and particles of granulosa distend the follicle.

tion method. A new sterile needle is used every time the needle tip passes through the vaginal mucosa. If the reaspirated flushing fluid is blood-tinged, a heparin-containing culture fluid is added to prevent clotting. Serration of the needle tip facilitates its visualization. After all the follicles have been aspirated, the pelvic organs are scanned to rule out active bleeding from puncture sites. Bacteriological cultures were collected from the vaginal vault before, and from the tip of the probe after, completion of the procedure.

The above-described technique was used in 123 patients, with an average of 3.6 oocytes recovered per procedure. Clinical pregnancies were achieved in 14 patients (11.4% per oocyte recovery). In the last series of 62 patients a 95.2% successful recovery rate was obtained, 3.82 oocytes per retrieval. Two hundred thirty-seven oocytes were recovered with a fertilization rate of 49%. In 59 patients (95%), embryo transfer was performed, and 10 pregnancies were achieved, 1 chemical and 9 clinical, for a 15.2% pregnancy rate relative to oocyte recovery as well as to embryo transfer. One single culture medium hosting one of the first recovered oocytes was infected. The cultures were sterile in the remaining cases.

We compared the last group of 47 patients who underwent laparoscopic oocyte retrieval with the last group of 62 patients who were chosen to undergo transvaginal oocyte recovery. Despite the fact that 6.2 oocytes were recovered per patient in the laparoscopic group, the pregnancy rates per retrieval and per embryo transfer in this group were 10.6 and 10.9%, respectively.

The transvaginal approach to follicular aspiration has several outstanding advantages over the transabdominal route:

1. The distance between the ovary and the probe is shorter transvaginally than by the transvesical route.
2. Higher-resolution images of the follicles are produced.
3. The distance traversed by the needle is shorter and there is less probability of bowel or blood vessel injury.
4. The procedure is quite painless and well tolerated by most of the patients, and recovery is quick.
5. The bladder is not entered; thus, any potential complication related to bladder injury is avoided.
6. There is no need for general or local anesthesia, significantly reducing complications and consequences of these procedures.
7. The procedure is significantly shorter by the transvaginal method.
8. The cost is significantly lower for the procedure, which can now be performed in a short-stay unit, eliminating operating room and recovery room expenses.

In summary, we consider the transvaginal approach useful in the follow-up and treatment of infertility in patients. The clarity of view of the pelvic organs and the ease of approach make transvaginal sonography the method of choice in most of these cases.

REFERENCES

1. Kratochwil A, Urban GV, Friedrich F: Ultrasonic tomography of the ovaries. Ann Chir Gynecol 1972;61:211–214.
2. Hackeloer BJ, Fleming R, Robinson HP: Correlation of ultrasonic and endocrinologic assessment of human follicular development. Am J Obstet Gynecol 1979;135:122–128.
3. Lenz S, Lauritsen JG, Kjellow M: Collection of human oocytes for in vitro fertilization by ultrasonically guided follicular puncture. Lancet 1981;1:1163–1164.
4. Feichtinger W, Kemeter P: Laparoscopic or ultrasonically guided follicle aspiration for in vitro fertilization. J In Vitro Fertil Embryo Transfer 1984;1(4):244–249.
5. Gleicher N, Friberg J, Fullan N, et al: Egg retrieval for in vitro fertilization by sonographically controlled vaginal culdocentesis. Lancet 1983;2:508–513.

6. Dellenbach P, Nisand I, Moreau L, et al: Transvaginal sonographically controlled ovarian follicle puncture for egg retrieval. Lancet 1984;1:1467–1471.
7. Hackeloer BJ, Robinson HP: Ultraschalldarstellung des wachsenden Follikels und Corpus luteum im normalen physiologischen Zyklus. Geb Frauenheilk 1978;38:163–168.
8. Hackeloer BJ: Ultrasound scanning of the ovarian cycle. J In Vitro Fertil Embryo Transfer 1984;1(4):217–220.
9. Baird DT, Fraser IS: Blood production and ovarian secretion rates of estradiol and estrone in women throughout the menstrual cycle. J Clin Endocrinol 1974;38:1009–1015.
10. De Cherney AH, Laufer N: The monitoring of ovulation induction using ultrasound and estrogen. Clin Obstet Gynecol 1984;27(4):993–1002.
11. Varygas JM, Marrs RP, Kletzki DA, et al: Correlation of ovarian follicle size and serum estradiol levels on ovulatory patients following clomiphene citrate for in vitro fertilization. Am J Obstet Gynecol 1982;144:569–573.
12. Siebel MM, McArdtle CR, Thompson IE, et al: The role of ultrasound in ovulation induction—A critical appraisal. Fertil Steril 1981;36:573–576.
13. De Crespigny L, O'Herlihy C, Robinson HP: Ultrasonic observation of the mechanism of human ovulation. Am J Obstet Gynecol 1981;139:616–640.
14. Smith B, Porter R, Ahuja K, et al: Ultrasonic assessment of endometrial changes in stimulated cycles in an in-vitro fertilization and embryo transfer program. J In Vitro Fertil Embryo Transfer 1984;1(4):233–238.
15. Feichtinger W, Kemeter P: Laparoscopic or ultrasonically guided follicle respiration for in vitro fertilization? J In Vitro Fertil Embryo Transfer 1984;1:244–249.
16. Feichtinger W, Kemeter P: Ultrasonically guided follicle aspiration as the method of choice for oocyte recovery for in vitro fertilization, in Proceedings of the Fourth World Congress on IVF, Melbourne. New York, Plenum Press, in press.
17. Kemeter P, Feichtinger W: Transvaginal oocyte retrieval using a transvaginal sector scan probe combined with an automated puncture device. Hum Reprod 1986;1(1):21–24.
18. Feichtinger W, Kemeter P: Ultrasound-guided aspiration of human ovarian follicles for in vitro fertilization, in Saunders RC, Hill M (ed): Ultrasound Annual 1986. New York, Raven Press, 1986, pp 25–37.
19. Cohen F, Debache C, Pez FP, et al: Transvaginal sonographically controlled ovarian puncture for oocyte retrieval for in vitro fertilization. J In Vitro Fertil Embryo Transfer 1986;3(5):309–313.

Index

V

Vaginal bleeding, 31, 108
Vaginal examination, one-finger, 24
Vaginal probe, physical considerations, 1–13, *See also* Probe
Velocity, 3, 3t
Ventricular system, lateral, 104
Vibrations, mechanical, 1

W

Wavelength, ultrasound, 2, 2f

Y

Yolk sac, 91f, 91, 94f, 94, 99f, 103f, 104f
  in abnormal pregnancy, 111, 120–121
  age at detection, 94, 98f
  relation to umbilical cord, 93f
  in tenth week, 100–104, 104f, 105f
"Yolk sac sign," 111
Yolk stalk, 93f

Z

Zone
  far, 8
  near, 8